CLINICS IN DEVELOPMENTAL MEDICINE NO. 107
QUADRUPLETS AND HIGHER MULTIPLE BIRTHS

Clinics in Developmental Medicine No. 107

QUADRUPLETS
and Higher Multiple Births

MARIE M. CLAY

University of Auckland
New Zealand

1989
Mac Keith Press
OXFORD: Blackwell Scientific Publications Ltd.
PHILADELPHIA: J. B. Lippincott Co.

©1989 Mac Keith Press
5a Netherhall Gardens, London NW3 5RN

All rights reserved. No part of this publication may be reproduced, stored in a retrieval system, or transmitted in any form or by any means, electronic, mechanical, photocopying, recording or otherwise, without the prior permission of the publishers

First published 1989

British Library Cataloguing in Publication Data

Clay, Marie M.
  Quadruplets and higher multiple births
  1. Man. Multiple birth.
  I. Title II. Series
  618.2'5

ISBN 978-0-521-41223-0

Printed in Great Britain at The Lavenham Press Ltd., Lavenham, Suffolk
Mac Keith Press is supported by **The Spastics Society, London, England**

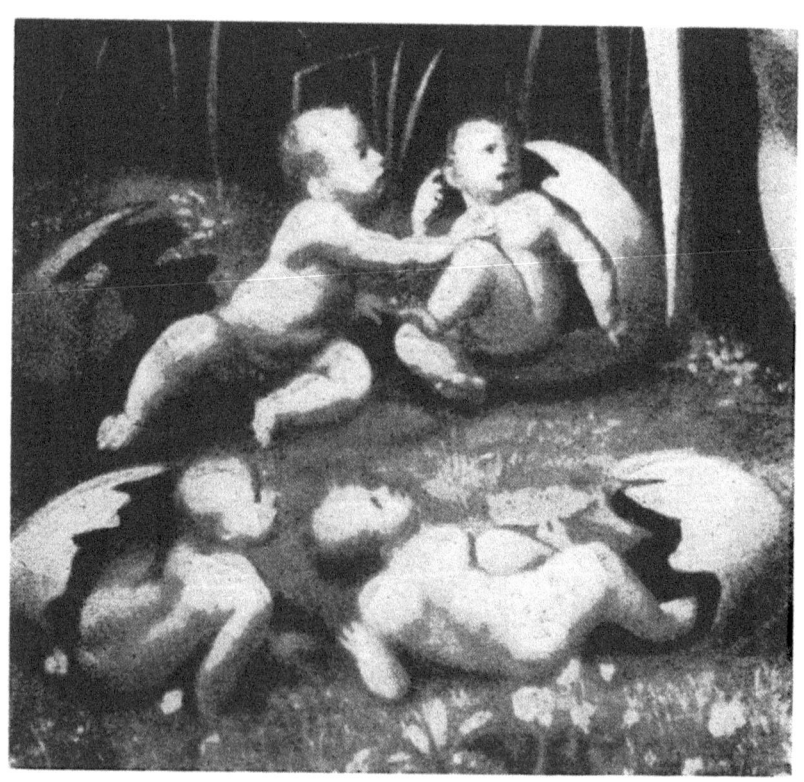

Detail from *Leda and the Swan* by Leonardo da Vinci

This book is dedicated to:

Jean Alexander (1929–1989)

– a mother of quadruplets –
whose questions convinced me
that there was a need for it

AUTHOR'S APPOINTMENTS

MARIE M. CLAY, DBE, PhD, MA(Hons), DipEd, FNZPsS, FNZEI

Professor of Education, University of Auckland, New Zealand.

CONTENTS

ACKNOWLEDGEMENTS	*page* x
FOREWORD *Elizabeth Bryan*	xi
FORENOTES	xii
1. INTRODUCTION	1
2. AN HISTORICAL CONTEXT	11
3. PREGNANCY AND BIRTH	30
4. FAMILY CONTEXT AND RELATIONSHIPS	35
5. STUDYING MULTIPLE SETS: OLD AND NEW DEVELOPMENTAL REPORTS	46
6. PSYCHOLOGY AND HIGHER MULTIPLE BIRTHS	76
APPENDICES	
1. Quadruplet births in the literature: a Catalogue of cases *Compiled by Marie M. Clay and Pat Chappelle*	95
2. Multiple birth associations, support groups and study centres	170
REFERENCES	174
INDEX	182

ACKNOWLEDGEMENTS

I would like to acknowledge the assistance I received from Mr Pat Chappelle and Dr Pamela Davies of the Mac Keith Press, in the extensive editing and preparation of this manuscript for publication; the friendship and help received from the parents of the Alexander quadruplets, and from the Johnson quadruplets; and the encouragement received in pursuing this project from Dr Barton MacArthur, Associate-Professor Ross Howie and Emeritus Professor Dennis Bonham.

FOREWORD

Professor Clay's book on quadruplets and higher multiples is very well timed. There has been a sudden and rapid increase in the number of such births due to the increasing and widespread use of new technologies for the treatment of infertility. In addition, more complete sets are surviving owing to improvements in neonatal care. The increase in numbers is likely to continue. We therefore need to know far more about these children.

Quads and quins have always attracted attention and interest but they have been the subject of very little systematic study. Most research workers have been daunted by the difficulties of collecting information on so rare a phenomenon. In contrast, however, Professor Clay was stimulated by her experience with a set of quadruplets to scour the literature with meticulous thoroughness. Her searches took her to obscure journals in many languages, as well as to the popular press (a useful source of information on higher multiples). The result is by far the richest compilation yet on the documentation of higher multiple births.

The book aims to provide a background for those wishing to study quads and quins, particularly the psychological aspects, and valuable methodological advice is given in the final chapter. However, research workers concerned with any aspect of the lives of multiple-birth children and their families will find this an enlightening and fascinating book.

Professor Clay gives helpful information on the biology of multiple births in general, enabling the reader to put these higher-order births into context. She sensitively describes many of the practical and emotional problems faced by families, which in themselves need further research. Her review complements the work undertaken by the British Study of Triplet and Higher Order Births (to be published Spring 1990).

The book provides innumerable fascinating personal stories but fully sustains its main purpose as an invaluable source of reference. It offers particular insights into the problems faced by families with quads and more and should be read by all those concerned with their care.

ELIZABETH BRYAN
MULTIPLE BIRTHS FOUNDATION
LONDON

FORENOTES

Catalogue of cases
Appended to this monograph is a 'Catalogue' of quadruplet birth case reports, from the mid-18th century up to the first recorded live delivery of quads conceived by means of *in vitro* fertilization. This list is as complete as an extensive search of the literature—conducted in the first instance by myself, and subsequently augmented by Pat Chappelle of the Mac Keith Press—has allowed. It is arranged in chronological order—where possible, of birth, or else of first report—and it is annotated with pertinent details and source references.

Confidentiality
Because public and media interest in higher multiple births often has proved overwhelming for the families involved, it is sometimes requested that no reports be made, or, where they are, that either the family should not be named or an assumed name be used. I have continued to respect this confidentiality, even where I have been able, in the course of my research, to establish the identity of subjects.

Metrification of birthweights
In most historical reports of multiple births, birthweights are given in imperial units (*i.e.* pounds and ounces). For this monograph, except where otherwise appropriate (*e.g.* in quotations), these have been converted to the metric equivalent, usually rounding up or down to the nearest five grams.

Multiple birth organizations
For the benefit both of future researchers and of parents of multiple sets, an international directory of multiple birth associations, support groups and study centres has been compiled by the Mac Keith Press, and is included as Appendix 2.

1
INTRODUCTION

In 1970 a set of quadruplets was referred to me at 3 years for well-baby checks on development: this seemed to provide a unique research opportunity. At that time they had only been talking for six months. Medical opinion was agreed that they were monozygotic*. What kind of research questions should one ask? What had been done in the past with such opportunities?

The questions were too complex for me to solve at the time. I completed the well-baby checks, made some controlled observations, participated in a language training programme at their kindergarten and monitored their slow but satisfactory progress in the first two years at school. After that there remained little reason for a developmental psychologist without a research purpose to be involved with their continued growth and development.

However, I became curious as to the effects of environment that might show up in children of identical heredity growing up differently in a set of home experiences which seemed so similar for each child. This was very different from the pervasive emphasis on heredity that existed in older and newer twin studies, and in the early studies of higher multiples.

In 1980, prompted by the frustration of this experience which seemed important but which I had not taken advantage of for scientific purposes, I began a literature search for studies of the growth and development of quadruplets, quintuplets and any larger sets. An early discovery maintained my confidence. It was Blatz's book, *The Five Sisters* (1939), which traced the preschool development of the famous Dionne quintuplets (the first surviving set of quins) to the age of 4 years. Journalistic accounts of their development have shaped public attitudes to other children of multiple births, with a shift from scientific wonder in the 1930s to a critical account of the 'melodrama' in the 1970s (Berton 1977). Developmental reports of higher multiple sets have been very rare; most were published between 1929 and 1944. It is as if the psychological study of higher multiple sets began and ended with the publication of Blatz's book. There has been little interest on the part of psychologists since that time.

A computer search of psychological abstracts from 1966 onwards produced almost no leads although there was an extensive literature on twins. Medical abstracts were more useful and it soon became clear that an historical study of older medical reports of multiple births would be needed. With the help of various cumulative indexes and several London libraries I began to locate older references.

My fascination with the topic grew as I realized that a massive shift in knowledge about plural pregnancies and births had taken place in the last 50 years after the birth of the Dionne quintuplets, paralleling dramatic shifts in techniques of monitoring pregnancy and establishing zygosity. I discovered that the first quads

*Abbreviated in text to MZ. (Similarly, DZ = dizygotic, TZ = trizygotic, QZ = quadrizygotic.)

surviving to adulthood, the Gehris (see pp. 13, 99–102), were born in 1880*, and that there were interesting insights into cultural attitudes in the historical literature even three centuries before that time. I caught up with the development of blood tests as a reliable aid to deciding whether babies are from one or more zygotes, and I was surprised to learn that there are potentially 22 different types of quadruplet sets if sex and zygosity are considered (Fig. 1.1), although for reasons which are not yet understood, there is a much greater preponderance of female quads and the all-male set is an extreme rarity (see Chapter 2, pp. 16–17).

Slowly I began to understand some of the reasons why knowledge about higher multiples was hard to find; one of those reasons lay in the keen interest shown by the public and responded to by the media.

Public interest

News of the birth of quadruplets, quintuplets or even higher multiple sets is of great interest to the public. Nichols (1950) believed that this interest was founded in a human fascination for all matters sexual and that this inspired the imaginative and fantastic stories about childbirth which occur in historical records. By the 1950s news of such cases was being systematically gathered and reported in the daily press all over the world. (The *New York Times Index (NYTI)* carries an annual listing of all the multiple births recorded in the world press for the year, and in my experience these records are reliable.) Higher multiple births occur rarely and to the public always appear exceptional. The births are newsworthy but the questions are of a superficial kind: How many sets of quins are there alive? What is the largest set ever born? How is that other set I heard about growing up?

The 1970s saw the arrival firstly of ovulation treatments for women otherwise unable to conceive, then of *in vitro* fertilization (IVF) techniques**. More higher multiple sets are born and survive today because of these treatments and because of the improvements in medical guidance and service to mothers and children. A media announcement of the arrival of a new multiple set rekindles public interest. However, after a brief update on some other previous sets, the interest slips away until the next announcement.

The babies, their families and doctors are photographed and quoted. Four or more children of precisely the same age and somewhat similar appearance are appealing subjects. Newspapers also respond with a series of pictures of other known sets—a birthday party, an outing or the first day at school are used as the most picturable indicators that the children are 'growing up'. One mother of quads complained to me, 'to some people we are the family peepshow'. Sameness and differences are also cause for comment, and the ups and downs of the family coping with multiples draw some sympathy. There is often an implied comment behind a birthday review article that it is surprising that the children grew normally to 10, 15

---

*Earlier reports exist in the literature (*e.g.* see pp. 96–97), but none of these can be considered to have been reliably authenticated.

**The first (surviving) set of quads conceived through IVF were born in Melbourne, Australia on 7 January 1984 (see Catalogue). The first surviving IVF quins were the Jacobssens (Alan, Brett, Connor, Douglas and Edward), born at the University College Hospital, London, on 26 March 1986. Their birthweights were all around 900g. (A report of their first birthday appeared in the *People* newspaper, 29 March 1987.)

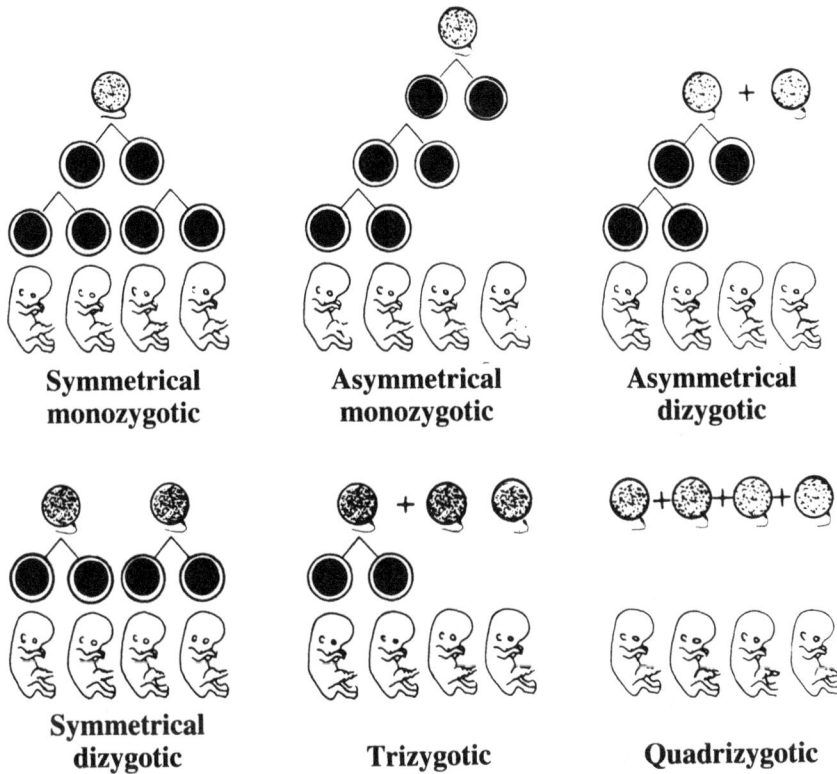

Fig. 1.1. Zygosity possibilities in quadruplet maternities (adapted from Hafez 1974).

or 20 years of age! Probably this public reminder about normality is a good thing.

Before it became common for the babies of a higher multiple gestation to be born alive the public interest focused on the mother, who would be visited even though her babies had died.

The mother, in spite of the crowds with which her chamber was continually filled, continued to recover . . (Garthshore 1787)

In 1935 the doctor attending a quadruplet birth in England reported:

Conditions were impossible in the cottage where they were born, and so I removed them to my house . . . where they could be better cared for and better protected from the public. (Harrison 1935)

Dr Allan Roy Dafoe concluded his notes on the birth of the Dionne quins (see p. 28) with the comment:

The publicity in connection with this case has been a serious problem and has caused me considerable trouble and worry. There has been no let-up from the moment of the uncle's naive enquiry to the North Bay paper as to how much it would cost to insert a birth notice for five babies born at one time. At first I resented what I felt was an intrusion into my private and professional affairs. Then I came to realize that I had no right to object to what had become a matter of continent-wide interest. (Dafoe 1934)

Today, interest in the higher multiple birth is apt to bring reporters, photographers and television crews flocking to the hospital, so an announcement will usually not be made until after the babies have been born and the hospital has made preparations for dealing with this interest. The main problems are that the hospital's normal and important routines may be disrupted and the patient's right to privacy infringed. If the mother and her family are opposed to this kind of publicity, it is the obligation of the hospital to avoid it (Fullerton *et al.* 1965). On the other hand, publicity can help in obtaining gifts and support for the family. Of course, the administrative or public relations department of a hospital can only develop a plan of action if they have advance warning of the event. Despite health care advances, hospitals and general practitioners are still taken by surprise on occasion by an unexpected higher multiple birth.

The problem of balancing public interest and family rights is well illustrated in this example from New Zealand in 1980. Born at between 5.00 and 5.30pm, the babies' pictures were in the following morning's papers and the nation knew their story. But the evening paper carried the headline, 'MUM YET TO SEE BABIES', clearly conveying to readers that the mother's rights had been pre-empted by a sensation-seeking press.

Media attention, if not carefully managed, can also have adverse effects on other family members, as illustrated in this quote from a magazine article on a family of quads (*You* in the *Mail on Sunday*, 8 July 1984):

'Every year on our birthday,' says Marie, 'we would be photographed by the newspapers . . . My mother used to think it was a nuisance because she preferred to stay in the background. And my father wanted us to stay a private family. Both my parents were very aware how much our [older] brother David felt left out. He was always pushed into the background when the photographers came to take pictures of us four. We felt very guilty about him. To this day he talks about it.'

Publicity is not always a problem. Some families have been at ease with it, as Gardner and Newman reported in three studies (1940*b*, 1942, 1943*a*). The Badgett quads, for instance, survived the initial publicity well:

When [they] were born they received a large amount of publicity. Like the Dionne quintuplets, they have regular scheduled hours for visitors. At first the babies were merely held up in front of a window to be viewed by spectators gathered in front of the house, but later on visitors were allowed to observe them as they played in the nursery. It is stated that at the end of the first year more than 500 persons per week had registered to see the quads at play. It has never been feasible to let the little girls play outdoors, for whenever it was attempted crowds soon gathered to watch them. (Gardner and Newman 1942)

A second study—of the Keys quadruplets born in 1916 and often in the public eye (Gardner and Newman 1940*b*)—suggests that they made an excellent adjustment to the interest shown in them:

[They] are probably the best known quadruplets in America. Their photographs have often appeared in the pictorial sections of our newspapers throughout the land. They have appeared in public on many occasions, chiefly as good-will ambassadors for the Oklahoma legislature. They have lived together until very recently when one of them was married. In spite of being quads and in spite of excessive publicity, they are as normal girls as one could find—happy and cheerful. In college they were always ready to cooperate with the student body or faculty in any enterprise. They were very much loved on the Baylor Campus.

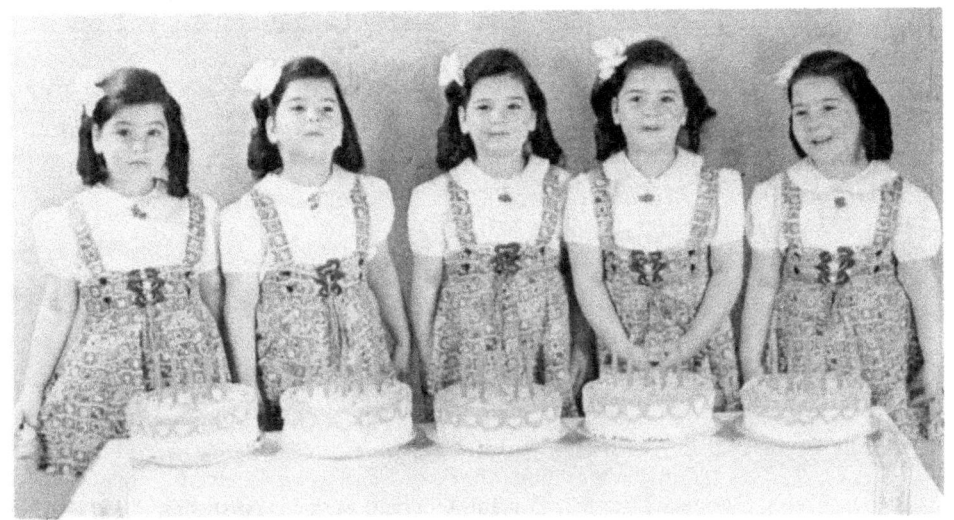

Fig. 1.2. The Dionne quintuplets (*l–r:* Emilie, Annette, Yvonne, Cecile, Marie) celebrating their fifth birthday (MacArthur and Dafoe 1939).

Since the arrival of fertility drugs a new and unfortunate kind of public reaction has been recorded in press interviews and medical reports. This is the abuse delivered to some families by those quick to judge and to criticize, as typified by this quote from a magazine article on a mother of quins (*Woman's Own*, 5 January 1980):

Complete strangers have come up to me in the park and called me names. "Disgusting woman," they've said. "How can you be so irresponsible?" Others have told me to get myself sterilised. Strangers, people I've never seen in my life before, demand intimate details of my medical history.

Individual differences in the parents' or children's ability to cope with this public interest must be respected. What may suit an outgoing family seeking interactions with people will be inappropriate for a quiet, self-sufficient family who value their privacy highly. The problem is that the first family is likely to gain materially from the public interest, though experience suggests only in minor ways, while the second family is allowed to struggle with little supplementation of its own resources.

The birth of the Dionne quintuplets at Corbeil, in the Callendar district of Ontario, in May 1934 stimulated enormous interest because no quins previously had survived more than 50 days. It is interesting to note that not only was the family offered advice by many members of the public but so too was their doctor (see plate overleaf). The interest in the Dionnes was exceptional (Schwesinger 1940), and to give them some protection they were made wards of King George VI and Queen Elizabeth. They were observed from behind a one-way screen by nearly two million visitors before their fifth birthday (Fig. 1.2). They had by that time amassed an estate worth three-quarters of a million dollars, and had brought employment and industry to a remote part of the Canadian hinterland.

SOME GOOD ADVICE?

Dr Allan Roy Dafoe was offered much advice by the general public on the management of his five young patients, the Dionne quintuplets. The range and level of this advice is illustrated by the following extract from one of his series of progress reports (Dafoe 1936).

I have learned a great deal in the last year and a half regarding infant care. My education has been further augmented through the medium of an international correspondence course in Medicine, Paediatrics, Bacteriology, and Therapeutics. My preceptors in this course have been varied, and included Christian Science followers, astrologers, chiropractors, veterinary surgeons, nurses, fathers, mothers, and maiden ladies. Many superstitious beliefs and ancient ideas regarding medicine and disease were passed along to me for my help. Letters containing advice and offers of help were received from Great Britain, India, Germany, France, Central America, Mexico, Australia, Philippine Islands, and from all over North America. I am quite sure that every milk preparation either 'in' or 'off' the market was mentioned in some of the letters. Goats and prize cows were offered to provide the necessary milk for the babies, and wet nurses made application for dairy appointments. It was suggested that a healthy lactating Yorkshire sow would solve our feeding problems. Her milk could either be obtained by pumping, or else preparing a place in the house whereby the babies could be directly suckled. It was intimated that the sow could be trained to adapt herself to this maternal duty. The reported onset of intestinal toxaemia produced an avalanche of letters, all of which contained suggested measures of treatment. Watermelon juice, infusions of blackberry root, horsetail plant, sassafras and knot weed were said to have produced spectacular results in similar cases. Whiskey was a common ingredient of many suggested remedies, and was to be used both internally and externally. The use of spirits, however, produced several letters of criticism for starting the children at such a tender age on a downward path. Sheep's dung tea, sweetened and warmed, was offered as a cure for 'The Blue Spells'. Placental blood in warm water was another secret imparted to me, for use in saving the babies. Of course, the usual letters containing messages from the stars, dreams of kidnapping, and warnings against poisoned food were plentiful. A beauty specialist, in her own words, 'a rather noted one', advised the use of her marvellous cream to remove the wrinkles from the premature babies. The contents of the morning mail offered great possibilities, and the following [is an example] from amongst the interesting communications received:

Dear Sir:

I notice by the evening paper that you are waiting on a lady who is mother of 5 girl babies. You sure have your hands full—What carries away babies is Diareh or summer complaint or looseness of the bowels—Now the best cure I know is perfectly harmless.

'Get pure Rye Whiskey and pour one teaspoon into a saucer. Take a clean pine sliver and set it on fire until it goes out. The dose for a medium cized baby (5–6 lbs) would be 1 drop, every 2 hrs. There ain't no poison in pure Rye Whiskey after it is burnt and I am anxious to see you pull through with them all. That is why I am putting you onto this cure.

(Signed) ....

However, this worldwide public interest in the Dionnes engendered strong feelings in some families against publicity of any kind. In extreme cases this has meant covering up all public evidence, and even distorting birth records by entering only a single birth. Often, no public or professional reporting of the event is allowed. In some cases, not knowing what scientists and reporters may do with the information they get and how this might rebound on the family, parents have reacted as the Dionne parents eventually did and have withdrawn the information from public availability. This introduces a bias in the knowledge we are able to get, and particularly in the reports in the press. (Medical professionals are more often trusted to make discreet reports.) This makes it difficult to check the authenticity of cases, and there has been one verified hoax (see p. 18) and others suspected from time to time in the press.

A more scientific interest
From these reports of the Dionnes it is possible to surmise some of the questions that were in the public mind. Probably they concerned child care and its relationship to growth and development. First came 'Can it be true?' and 'Will they live?', and then, as the reports of physical care and development seemed to confirm that they would, 'Will they grow up to be normal human beings?'. Schwesinger (1940) attributed some of this public interest in the Dionnes to 'educational curiosity'. She wrote:

The material changes in the Callendar landscape brought about by the business expansion are insignificant as compared with the stimulation which the Callendar experiment is giving to a constantly watching world in bringing home a realization that continuous right care and supervision should not only develop bigger and better babies but should also mould more wholesome and charming personalities.

Of what scientific interest were the Dionne quintuplets to scientists of the day? Schwesinger discussed two questions:

1. What are the possibilities and limits of mental and physical development through maximal opportunity and the best possible kind of rearing at least insofar as we can determine what these most favorable influences are? The answer to this question becomes the concern of parents, educators, eugenists, psychologists and child specialists everywhere.
2. The second question of major importance to science is how much variation in traits will appear when five identically similar organisms are reared in the one highly controlled environment? The answer to this question will throw its quota of light on the much thrashed at hereditary–environment problem.

The first question reflected the public's concern in the 1930s and '40s about the relationship of child-rearing to later outcome. It was debated in the popular and scientific press as reports of the Dionnes came to hand, and later discussants have been quick to seize upon the personal stories of the girls* to reflect negatively on multiple rearing in general or the Dionnes' routines in particular.

The present volume was prepared in the belief that more research needs to be

---

*The Dionnes' stories are poignantly related in the book *We Were Five* (1965), co-authored by James Brough and the four surviving 'quints' (the fifth sister, Emilie, having died in 1954), and further described in Berton's 1977 monograph *The Dionne Years: A Thirties Melodrama*. (See also p. 27.)

done with children from higher multiple sets, and in particular quadruplets. It seemed important to make available in one place, to any person whose profession brings them into contact with such children, the main points from the small literature which exists, but which takes time and effort to find. Schwesinger's second point, concerning environment and its effect on learning sequences, has never been investigated in any systematic way: such a study, among higher order sets with MZ members, would be a useful one for psychologists to take up. Methodological issues are discussed in Chapter 6.

Prospects for renewed scientific interest
Co-twin studies were under way in the 1930s in Moscow and Yale. Then in 1934 the Dionne quins arrived, stimulating the scientific world to greater activity. Child-rearing variables were manipulated in various ways. Yet by 1940 science had lost its window on this group following the parents' irrevocable decision to end its involvement with outsiders. Perhaps science, unlike general medical practice, forgot to take some human variables into account. The study of the Dionnes ended. Co-twin studies began to be criticized as developmental psychology changed fashion in theories and strengthened its methodologies and its interpretative logic.

Meanwhile medical researchers continued more than a century of work on incidence figures, and more evidence was produced on the timing and types of twinning processes and multiple pregnancies. Better zygosity indicators were sought and found as blood-typing became more refined. Geneticists studying the interactions of heredity and experience maintained an interest in the intelligence and personality of twins. Psychologists' interest has remained with the larger-scale studies of twins for two reasons—resources and funding have helped locate research samples, and computers have made feasible more complex analyses of hereditary and environmental influences and their interaction.

Medical science gave a new burst of energy to the subject when the treatment of women with fertility drugs began in the 1960s. This brought about an increase in the incidence of quadruplet, quintuplet, sextuplet and septuplet gestations. Survival of a higher multiple set was now a strong possibility (Schenker *et al.* 1981). Further interest was generated in 1984, when the world's first quadruplets conceived through IVF were born in Melbourne.

Today, improved prenatal and neonatal care has succeeded in keeping six babies alive from one pregnancy. The medical profession has, over decades, profited from the careful recording of plural births and the characteristics of the early years of development, in records that go back at least to 1566. But we still need a better understanding of the influences on the development of children from plural births and of their particular educational and psychological needs.

Children of multiple sets offer several research possibilities to the professional involved with the children and their families. These professionals may be doctors, nurses, psychologists, social workers, teachers or preschool workers. In the course of their work it would be appropriate for them to plan their record-keeping (with due regard to permissions and professional ethics) so that other professionals and families of higher multiples can benefit from their observations. Illustrative research approaches might be as follows.

* Records would be kept by the hospital in such a way that data could be accumulated across a series of cases even if personnel and/or techniques changed over the course of the series.
* Records might be collected before educational transitions such as a change of school, and regular checks made of changes that occur over some suitable time period.
* Any training intervention could be designed to make note of changes in behaviour, and the similarities or differences observed across the set.
* Any records of medical appraisals or interventions should include accounts of the developmental aspects of performance, reactions, relationships and environmental factors wherever possible.

These suggestions stem from the fact that this is a very small minority population and information needs to be contributed by whichever professionals have the opportunity to work with the children. A lack of access to the children's earlier records should not deter the observer or researcher from making a careful contribution to knowledge, with the one proviso that every attempt should be made to answer the important question of zygosity (see Chapter 3, pp. 32–34).

The unusual degree of control over many variables that is possible with higher multiples makes them important research subjects. (An analogy is with the study of certain single adults with known neurological trauma, whose records contribute greatly to our understanding of how the brain works.) With higher multiples the research design opportunity comes from the possibility of comparing individuals of similar and different zygosity status, and also being able to achieve some manageable control over environmental variables, especially those in the home.

Because of the low incidence of quadruplets, the field psychologist rather than the research psychologist is the one most likely to come into contact with the family through referral by an interested general practitioner, a perplexed family seeking help in child management from the local psychological service, or a school anxious to provide for the children's best interests but overawed by the exceptionality of the case. It is likely that educational, child or clinical psychologists have been asked to carry out well-baby checks from time to time on multiple sets, and that this has been done but without any commitment on the part of the psychologist to continuing documentation of the children's growth and development. Interest is usually focused on helping the children to maintain a normal set of achievements and a happy adjustment in the face of rather unusual pressures in their lives.

Most physicians and psychologists go through their professional lives without seeing a multiple set comprising more than two children. However, if the opportunity should come their way, I would encourage them to accept a long-term case study assignment for as long a period as is consistent with the willingness of the children and their family to co-operate. By approaching the problem as scientific study and using their own particular strengths and interests they could study the range of variability that can be induced in phenotypes (a) controlled by genetic factors, or (b) not simply or tightly controlled by such factors. Results should be reported if possible, and editors of journals need publication policies that will allow bodies of knowledge on such highly variable and low incidence groups to be built up. Otherwise knowledge about them disappears and bias in attribution emerges.

Communication problems
There are communication difficulties in this area of study aside from the publication questions raised above for anyone who wants information, be they reporter, parent, medical practitioner or researcher. Important issues are the authentication of the existence of multiple sets; confidentiality of records and reports; rarity of books and sources which go quickly out of print and disappear; low incidence of subjects; differences across academic disciplines; language barriers; and parental reactions to the birth and to public or scientific interest. Some of my encounters will illustrate these problems.

★ Mayer's (1952a,b) scholarly history of reference to plural births of six, seven or more children reaches back through art, literature and historical documents of many countries. It illustrates clearly the problems of authentication of historical cases and the importance of medical reports that have been preserved.

★ Sometimes the only record of a multiple birth was in an obscure journal with few existing copies. Many times my research came to a dead end. Exploring the mechanized stacks of the British Medical Association Library I was delighted to find copies of *Semana Medicala*, only to discover that a particular issue I needed was not among the delicate, brown-with-age volumes in the stacks.

★ There are communication problems across language and scientific disciplines. A 1974 report on a Polish male quadruplet set (the 'Wroclaw quads'—see Catalogue, 25 October 1954) claimed they were unique as the only MZ set alive, when in fact there were three other living sets recorded in the English literature, though these were all female. Or did the translator perhaps miss the 'only *male* set' somewhere in the article?

★ Even an author's respect for the confidentiality of information presents a reviewer of the literature with problems. The obstetrician, the serologist, the paediatrician and the psychologist might each publish a report in the journals of their respective disciplines which preserves the identity of the family in different ways. How is the reviewer to know whether s/he is dealing with one, two, three or four different sets?

There are insufficient records concerning the growth and development of higher multiple sets to overcome the difficulties of interpreting data influenced by so many biological and environmental variables. The lack of publicly verifiable information has led to the persistence of a public and professional belief that exceptionality precludes normality for multiple set children (even though reports are more usually made of healthy intact sets than of those with disabled members, unless the developmental outcome is a success story as in the case of the Wroclaw quads). It is crucial that doubts about normality be laid to rest, if only because their persistence adversely affects the upbringing and educational opportunities of these children.

It is important, as we venture further into applications of genetic counselling, artificial fertilization techniques and perhaps in the future human genetic manipulation of even a minor kind, that more information of better quality be available than that which I have been able to collate in this volume, so that individuals might have some basis for making their choices about the implications of rearing a higher multiple set of children.

2
AN HISTORICAL CONTEXT

Studies of incidence
Human multiple births are comparatively rare. Hellin (1895) suggested that a mathematical relationship existed between the occurrence of twins, triplets and higher multiple gestations. Working from South German statistics he concluded that the frequency of triplets would be approximately the square of the frequency of twins. His prediction for the occurrence of twins was 1:89 and for triplets $1:89^2$. He thought that the incidence of quadruplets should be the frequency of twins to the third power, $1:89^3$. These predictions were checked by Greulich (1930) on over 121 million births in 21 nations between 1915 and 1925 and his figures for actual cases were surprisingly close to Hellin's—twins occurred 1:85.2, triplets $1:87.3^2$, and quadruplets $1:87.5^3$. A second check by Guttmacher (1953) produced similar figures for 57 million births in the USA from 1928 to 1949. Guttmacher claimed that these rates of occurrence should be regarded as a mathematical approximation calculated as follows:

If the twinning frequency of a population is expressed as $1/N$ then the triplet frequency is $1/N^2$ and the quadruplet frequency is $1/N^3$.

Modifications to this formula have been proposed by authors who sought to rectify two omissions in Hellin's argument: the lack of distinction between the different types of triplets and quadruplets, and the variation which occurs with maternal age (Allen and Firschein 1957, Bulmer 1958, Allen 1960). Over the past 20 years treatments of infertile women have introduced an unpredictable factor into such incidence studies.

Racial variations
Studies have shown that there are consistent differences in the frequencies of multiple births among different races. Multiple gestations generally have the highest incidence among Black populations (Hamlett 1935; Nylander 1969, 1971, 1975) and the lowest among Oriental groups (Gedda 1961), with Caucasian stock in an intermediate position. For example Nylander (1971) found unusually high multiple-birth rates among the Yoruba people of Western Nigeria where the twinning rate was four times that of Caucasian rates in the UK and USA, and the triplet rate 16 times as high. On the other hand Imaizumi and Inouye (1979) reported a twinning rate for Japanese births from 1951 to 1968 of only one per 156 deliveries. These racial variations apply only to DZ twinning. The incidence rates for MZ twinning seem to be constant across countries and races, at about one per 200 to 300 births.

Browne and Dixon (1978) published a summary of predictions for multiple births among Caucasians, giving figures of one in 80 for twins, one in 8000 for triplets and one in 350,000 for quadruplets, with quintuplets recorded at least 40 times and sextuplets seven times. Documented variations from country to country were explained by both genetic and environmental factors. A secular decline in twinning rates from the early 1950s until the 1970s has been observed almost worldwide, largely confined to DZ twinning (Murphy and Botting 1989). Botting *et al.* (1987) reported a reduction in the twinning rates in England and Wales between 1960 and 1983 from about one in 80 to one in 100 (in contrast, however, the rate for quadruplet births has virtually doubled in that time—see below). Hamlett's (1935) figures for the USA showed that both Black and Caucasian incidence rates were lower than predicted for triplets and higher than predicted for quadruplets.

Many estimates of multiple birth rates were made during the 19th century, derived from large numbers of actual births. For example, Wappaus (1859, reported by Dahlberg 1926) recorded statistics on 19 million births in Middle Europe; while Jenkins (1927) republished data from Veit (no ref. given) on 13 million births in Prussia from 1826 to 1849, from Prinzing (1892) on 63 million births in Germany from 1871 to 1880, and from Neefe (1877) on a set of 50 million births. Veit, Prinzing and Neefe reported quadruplet birth rates ranging from $1:72^3$ to $1:92^3$; Prinzing's data yielded 114 quadruplet births over the decade covered (a rate of approximately $1:81^3$). On the other hand, a somewhat higher incidence of just over $1:62^3$ obtains from figures quoted by Brattström (1914) for the 16 million births recorded in Sweden between 1751 to 1910.

These data indicate a much higher incidence rate for quadruplet births than would be indicated by the small number of authenticated reports available in published sources. Few babies survived the neonatal period; no higher multiple sets surviving intact past the neonatal period are reported before 1847*. These early studies reflect the curiosity that existed in the scientific community of the time about the rare and largely unexplained phenomena of multiple gestations.

Changes in incidence rates

Based on a study of the multiple birth rates in Sweden from 1794 onwards and in Finland from 1859, Eriksson *et al.* (1976) concluded that there had been a decline over time. The rates for triplets and quadruplets in those countries were three to four times as high in the 18th century as they are today. In terms of Hellin's approximation, quadruplet maternities were higher than expected up to the middle of the 19th century and lower during this century.

Falls in (DZ) twinning rates since 1918 have also been reported in England, Scotland and Wales, Hungary, the Netherlands, Poland, the USA and many other countries (James 1972). During this period the average family size has been shrinking and a woman's child-bearing years have been shortened. As the chances of a mother giving birth to twins or other multiples increase with age and with the number of her previous pregnancies (Scheinfeld 1973, Nylander 1975), the fall in multiple birth rates is not surprising. Eriksson *et al.* (1976), however, do not attribute it to social and cultural variables alone. They suggest that trends in maternal age and parity occur alongside other changes such as the erosion of

---

*See, however, the case of Feodor Vassilyev (pp. 96–97).

cultural and national isolation and marriage migration patterns. The effect has been to change the proportion of MZ twins among all twins in the US population from 30.7 per cent in 1918 to 36.7 per cent in 1958 (Scheinfeld 1973).

In recent years there has been an increase in the incidence of higher multiple births as a result of advances in medical science. First came the administration of fertility drugs to women with ovulatory failure: superovulation leading to higher multiple births has been one of the more common complications of this treatment, occurring in an estimated 5 to 20 per cent of pregnancies depending on the drugs used, the historical period surveyed and the sample studied (Gemzell 1967, Ellis and Williamson 1975, Wyshak 1978). These multiple pregnancies are considered undesirable because of an increased risk of ante- and perinatal loss (Jewelewicz 1975), and methods are under trial aimed at averting this complication. There is a general consensus that multiple pregnancies in such cases are multiovular. In the 1980s the techniques known as IVF (*in vitro* fertilization) and GIFT (gamete intra-fallopian transfer) have been mainly responsible for the increase in higher multiple births.

The incidence of quadruplets

The earliest (authenticated) case that I could find in the literature of a set of quads all born alive and surviving the neonatal period was that reported by Leopold (1871). Born in Germany in 1847, one died of bronchial pneumonia at 1½ years, one of scarlet fever at 7 years, a third of typhus at 20 years, and at the time of Leopold's report the fourth was still living. The first set to survive intact to adulthood were the Gehris, two boys and two girls born in Switzerland in 1880 (Glaser 1881) and studied retrospectively by Schlaginhaufen (1940) when they were 60 years of age (Fig. 2.1). Lachmann (1907) reported the delivery of quads of a quite remarkable total birthweight of 11,750g, all said to be well-nourished and thriving, though no further report was found. In a chronology of survivors the next report was from a midwife in Boston, Massachusetts, of the birth in 1912 of four girls, all surviving at 4 months but with no further report. Pinard (1920) reported the birth in 1915 of quadruplets in France. One died in an accident at the age of 16 years; the other three were still alive at 33 (Vaudescal *et al.* 1948). A set who survived to adulthood and whose development was reported extensively were the Keys quads, four girls born in Oklahoma in 1915 (Spier 1928, Brintle 1931, Gardner and Newman 1940). These cases indicate that survival and development for full sets of quadruplets first became a possibility in the years spanning the turn of the century.

Since then, studies in various countries have determined the incidence of quadruplet births as follows:
- ★ in the USA, 114 sets born between 1915 and 1948 (Nichols 1952), and 27 sets between 1947 and 1954 (Allen and Firschein 1957);
- ★ in Canada, four sets born between 1945 and 1948 (Stocks 1952);
- ★ in England and Wales, 29 sets born between 1931 and 1951 (McKeown and Record 1953), and 112 sets between 1952 and 1988 (see Table 2.I);
- ★ in Japan, 32 sets born between 1951 and 1968 (Imaizumi and Inouye 1979);
- ★ in New Zealand, eight sets (live-)born between 1960 and 1989 (*personal data*).

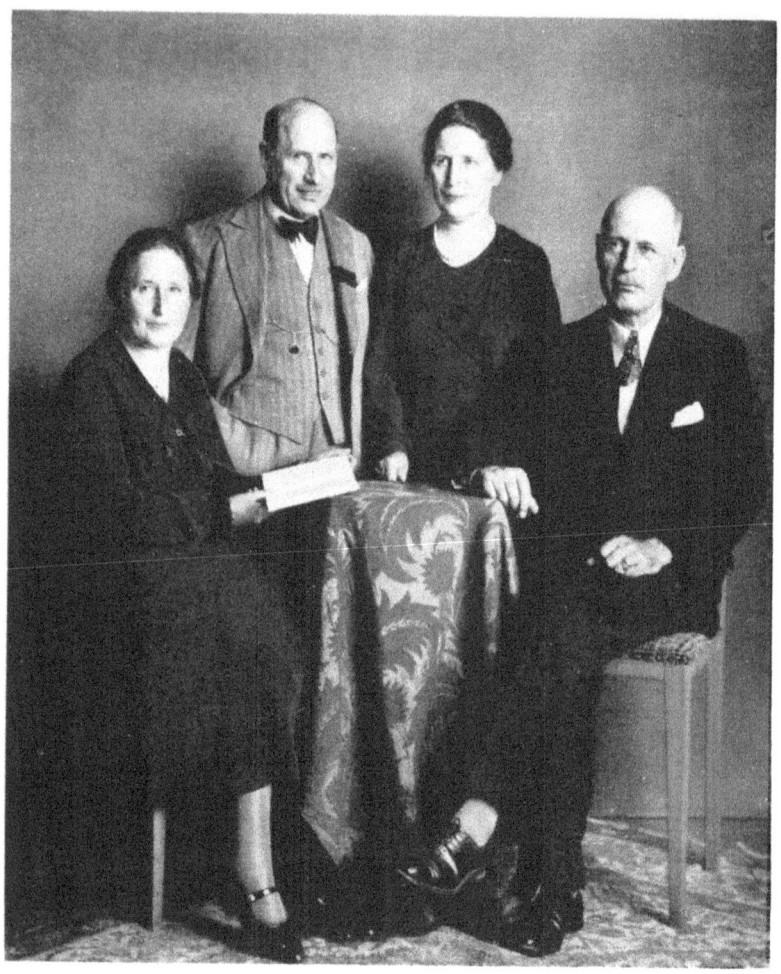

Fig. 2.1. The Gehri quads (*l–r:* Bertha, Arthur, Rosa and Oskar), photographed a few weeks before their 60th birthday (Schlaginhaufen 1940).

For any particular country, the number of surviving sets will depend upon the annual birth rate, the incidence of multiple births for the ethnic groups of that country, and the conditions of prenatal, natal and postnatal care. A developmental or educational psychologist interested in estimating surviving sets would have to allow for infant mortality figures for multiple births. There might be as many as 40 quadruplet sets in the schools of the USA in any one year, and they would comprise a sizeable potential study group of 160 children. It is only in countries with small populations or low levels of maternity care that the surviving quadruplet set is still today comparatively rare.

Any study of sets in a particular age band would have to be carried out cross-nationally to build up numbers, and that would be complicated by linguistic and cultural differences. A further complication would be the variety of types with respect to zygosity (see Fig. 1.1, p. 3).

There are well-documented medical records of many multiple pregnancies which did not result in viable births. Babies are lost from such pregnancies at much higher rates than from singleton conceptions. This is due to malformations arising early in fetal development, stillbirths at a rate three times as high as that for singletons, and neonatal deaths, often due to preterm birth, at seven times the singleton rate (Potter 1963). Quadruplets and higher multiples have less chance of surviving as intact sets than twins or triplets. Guttmacher (1953) pointed out that the vital statistics of all nations recorded only viable births and not total pregnancies, and that this produces a consistent error in the statistics for multiple gestations. Nor are the figures for spontaneous abortions or previable terminations of multiple pregnancies included in national calculations. For example, in the United States from 1948 to 1958, 42 quadruplet births were recorded, whereas the Hellin approximation (see p. 11) would predict 45. A count of gestations rather than viable births might make up the difference or might even produce a large discrepancy over and above that figure.

Scheinfeld (1968) summarized the trends as follows:

.. medical advances are enabling a greater proportion of supertwins to be born and to stay alive. On the other hand, the decrease in child-bearing by mothers in the supertwinning brackets (older mothers, with many previous pregnancies) should be causing a drop in supertwin conceptions. Upsetting this balance, however, may be the increased production in supertwinning as a result of the new hormone treatments. Whether, and to what extent, the latter factor will result in a bumper crop of supertwins in the years ahead may depend largely on how many women are eager to give birth to a whole family at one time.

Figures for all maternities registered in England and Wales are compiled annually by the Office of Population Censuses and Surveys; data for the years 1952 to 1988 are reproduced in Table 2.I. Over this whole 36 year period 112 quadruplet sets were registered out of a total of just over 26 million births, giving an overall incidence rate of around $1:62^3$. However, a breakdown of these data reveals a sharp increase in the rate from $1:94^3$ in the years 1952–1970, to $1:53^3$ in the decade 1971–1980, and $1:45^3$ from 1982 to 1988.

SEX RATIO

The ratio of females to males increases as the number of children born in one confinement increases. Based on data from the US Bureau of the Census (1942), including 99 sets of quads born between 1920 and 1942, Walker (1947) calculated the following ratios:

★ singletons   ... 94 girls per 100 boys;
★ twins   ... 97 girls per 100 boys;
★ triplets   ... 101 girls per 100 boys;
★ quadruplets ... 107 girls per 100 boys.

Adding data from Canada, Australia, New Zealand, South Africa, England and Wales, the ratio for quads rose to 112:100. A much higher figure of 156:100, based on US data from the Metropolitan Life Assurance Co. (1944) covering the years 1933–1941, is sometimes quoted; however, that ratio reflects an unusual spate of female quad births in three consecutive years during that period (Walker 1947).

TABLE 2.I
Maternities with multiple births in England and Wales from 1952 to 1988*

Year	All maternities	Twins	Triplets	Quadruplets	Quintuplets	Sextuplets	Septuplets
1952	680,715	8,525	64	1			
1953	691,180	8,703	83		1		
1954	681,058	8,655	69				
1955	675,026	8,437	87	1			
1956	707,921	8,660	78	1			
1957	730,524	9,273	95	3			
1958	747,536	9,287	90				
1959	755,294	8,934	87				
1960	791,584	9,086	77				
1961	817,271	9,570	82	1			
1962	844,265	9,756	88	1			
1963	858,884	9,960	100				
1964	880,173	10,135	99	4			
1965	866,713	9,695	79				
1966	853,481	9,418	82	1			
1967	835,433	9,117	68	2			
1968	822,247	8,697	84	1		1	
1969	799,763	8,259	79	1	1	1	
1970	786,587	8,042	100	1			
1971	784,899	8,000	69	3	2		
1972	726,715	7,345	81	3	2		
1973	677,125	6,615	71	2			
1974	640,777	6,151	60	4			
1975	603,666	5,909	72	7			
1976	584,263	5,538	76	4	2	1	
1977	569,073	5,449	68	2			
1978	595,515	5,859	62	8	1		
1979	636,884	6,099	76	6			
1980	654,501	6,308	91	4	1		
1981**	632,350						
1982	623,511	6,201	70	6			
1983	626,277	6,293	89	4		1	
1984	633,965	6,321	80	5			
1985	653,142	6,700	93	7	2	1	
1986	657,308	6,969	123	10	2	1	
1987	677,467	7,186	125	7	1		1
1988	689,153	7,452	157	12	1		

*Based on Office of Population Censuses and Surveys data (OPCS 1984; Table 6.1), with additional information courtesy of the Study of Triplets and Higher Order Births (*personal communication*) and the OPCS Fertility Statistics Unit (*personal communication*—1988 data used by permission). Figures include maternities with one or more stillbirths.
**Breakdowns for 1981 are not available due to industrial action by local registrars of births and deaths in that year. The overall figure was extrapolated from a 10 per cent sample.

Analysis of those 167 sets of quads included in the Catalogue (Appendix 1) for whom the sex of all four members is known yields a breakdown of 373 females and 295 males (a ratio of approximately 126:100). Table 2.II indicates the composition of these quad sets by sex. It can be seen that all-male sets are comparatively uncommon, and, somewhat surprisingly, that the 'ideal' combination of 'two of each' is the most frequently occurring (over 28 per cent of cases).

The reason for this female preponderance has not yet been satisfactorily

TABLE 2.II

Composition by sex of quadruplet sets included in the Catalogue of cases (Appendix 1)*

Female	Male	N	%
4	—	38	22.8
3	1	33	19.8
2	2	47	28.1
1	3	28	16.8
—	4	21	12.6

*Breakdown includes only those cases for whom the sex of all four quads is known (N = 167).

explained, though some authors (*e.g.* Stocks 1952) have suggested that it 'may be due to a greater tendency for male embryos to die at an early stage of pregnancy (producing an abortion) when the pregnancy is multiple than when it is single'.

Five and more

This volume addresses itself primarily to quadruplets but brief comment on multiple sets of five or more is needed at some points.

From time to time through history—in literature, folklore, art, and in medical and municipal records—there have been accounts of more than five children born at one time to the same mother. Ignorance of the origins of multiple gestations has in the past made life difficult for these mothers. 'Wonderbirths' were often regarded as punishments for adultery. In two fascinating articles Mayer (1952a,b) tried to tease fact from fiction and establish the authenticity of these early reports. His first article dealt with accounts of sextuplet births and the second covered higher multiples.

The highest plural birth since Mayer's review and reported in both the press and medical literature is nine—four girls and five boys—born at the Royal Hospital for Women in Sydney, Australia (*NYTI** 1971, Carey 1976). Two were stillborn; seven were born alive but none lived beyond 7 days. It was thought that they were from nine separate ova. The following year there were press reports of another set of nine children in Pennsylvania, none surviving (*NYTI* 1972).

Newspaper reports cannot always be relied upon as the only source of evidence of a multiple birth. The most celebrated hoax (see plate overleaf) was an announcement of octuplets. I located two references to the birth of octuplets in press reports that were not matched by reports in the medical literature. Four boys and four girls were born two months preterm in Mexico City, none surviving (*NYTI* 1967), and from the birth of three boys and five girls in Naples, two were reported as leaving hospital (*NYTI* 1979).

Turksoy *et al.* (1967) reported a set of septuplets, one stillborn at home and six previable babies delivered in hospital and dying shortly after birth. They were of little more than 4 months gestational age. It appeared to the authors that seven ova had been fertilized.

*New York Times Index.

THE OCTUPLET SQUIB – THE GREAT HOAX OF 1872

The most celebrated hoax among the stories of multiple births concerns octuplets and was fully reported by Mayer (1952*b*, pp. 256–258):

Eunice Mowery who lived in Trumbull County, Ohio State, had a suitor, a printer by occupation, whom she rebuffed in favour of Timothy Bradlee. In 1872, when the girl apparently became Mrs Bradlee, the jilted printer wanted to get even with her. Hence on the night of August 20 to 21, he broke into the offices of a local newspaper at Warren, Ohio (East of Cleveland, not far south of Lake Erie), and removed a block of type from the first page of next morning's paper, and inserted in its place his squib about Mrs Bradlee. He struck off 20–30 copies with the story of octuplets, then he reset the local paper in its original form. The spurious issues he dispatched to various daily papers in the Eastern U.S., and the story with the octuplets was reprinted several times during August and September of 1872 both in the daily newspapers and in the various scientific and medical magazines.

Here is what the jilted suitor printed. On 21 August, 1872, Mrs Timothy Bradlee, Trumbull Co., Ohio, gave birth to 8 children, 3 girls and 5 boys. They are all living and healthy, but quite small. She was married six years previously when, on the day of her marriage, she weighed 273 lbs. She has given birth to two pairs of twins, making 12 children in six years. She herself was a triplet, her mother and father also both having been twins, and her grandmother one of five pairs of twins. Quite an elaborate chain of lies!

I do not know the number of dailies and weeklies which picked up the story first. One of the earliest was the Cincinnati-Lancet for August, 1872, from which it was taken over by the Columbus Democrat for September, 1872, published at Columbus, Wisconsin.

In the September 26, 1872, issue of the Boston Medical and Surgical Journal there were 12 and a half lines devoted in the "Medical Miscellany" column to the narrative of the Ohio octuplets, and the Medical Times and Gazette also carried the same faked report. It was also repeated by Foy in 1890, and by many such works as the one written by Gould and Pyle in 1897 on the Anomalies and Curiosities of Medicine.

On March 24, 1914, Dr G. H. Parker, of Cambridge, Massachusetts, became curious about the Bradlee octuplets in Ohio and sent a letter of inquiry to the County Clerk of Trumbull County for further details. The Clerk of Courts, Mr M. B. Tayler, wrote to Parker on 30 March, 1914 that there was no truth in the report on the Trumbull County octuplets and it was the work of a practical joker. Parker published the clerk's letter in Science, and wrote to the Editor of the Boston Medical & Surgical Journal who then corrected the 1872 misstatement.

The 'squib' was reprinted in many daily papers in the United States and in a number of medical magazines. It took nearly half a century to detect the hoax.

Two years later a well-documented case of septuplet conception was reported (Aiken 1969, Cameron *et al.* 1969). The babies were delivered by caesarian section at 32 weeks. Six were born alive, of whom one died within the hour and two more at 12 and 20 days. The seventh had stopped developing much earlier in the pregnancy and was delivered as a *fetus papyraceus**.

Burnell (1974) reported a mother's reaction to the loss of septuplets (see Chapter 4, p. 36). Prior to conception she had been on a course of menotropins. Right up until the time of the birth, only triplets had been expected. Two of the babies were anencephalic, and none survived longer than 12 hours.

Two further sets of septuplets have been reported in the press, both conceived as a result of fertility drug treatments. The first case occurred in May 1985 in California (*NYTI* 1985). The babies were delivered 12 weeks preterm by caesarian section; one was stillborn, the others weighed between 480 and 825g. All died within a few days. The second set were born in Liverpool's Oxford Street hospital in August 1987, 17 weeks preterm, again by caesarian section. The birthweights ranged from 425 to 735g. All were liveborn but none survived beyond a few days (*Daily Mail*, 1 September 1987).

Mayer (1952*a*) noted several reports of sextuplets. There was a well-documented case in Italy in 1888 when the wife of a village mayor gave birth to four boys and two girls, none of whom survived; and in 1903 a native woman in Accra, Ghana (known then as the Gold Coast) bore five boys and a girl, none living past 4 days (an illustration of the first case and a photograph of the latter were reproduced in Mayer's article).

Nichols (1954) gave a detailed account of the Bushnell sextuplets, born in Chicago in September 1866. All six children—three boys and three girls—were born alive; two died in infancy but the others survived to adulthood, the next dying at 68 years. *Look* magazine of 25 October 1938 published photos of the three surviving members, and in the same year they were featured by Robert Ripley, creator of the *Believe It Or Not* series, in one of his New York radio broadcasts. The last survivor, Mrs Alincia Bushnell Parker, died in March 1952, aged 88, an obituary sketch being published in the Rochester *Times-Union* of March 27th**. Nichols also gave details of an unusual case of six at one birth which occurred in Missouri in 1936. A 36-year-old mother gave birth at term to a healthy baby girl, followed a few minutes later by five diminutive fetuses of around 2 to 3 months gestational age and enclosed in a separate amniotic sac. The immature 'quin' set apparently were the result of a superfetation, or later impregnation, and might well have proceeded to viability had their development not been interrupted by the living daughter's birth.

In 1974 Gutowitz *et al.* reported a successful sextuplet pregnancy in South Africa, with three boys and three girls born in optimal physical health. The authors stated that the babies had remained *in utero* longer than most multiples, and had a

---

*A *fetus papyraceus* (or *fetus compressus*) occurs in a multiple pregnancy when one fetus dies and becomes flattened out between the remaining, developing fetus(es) and the uterine wall.

**The mother, Mrs Jennie Bushnell, is also reputed to have previously borne triplets, deceased within eight months; and subsequently, another set of triplets and, sometime after 1870, quintuplets, none surviving.

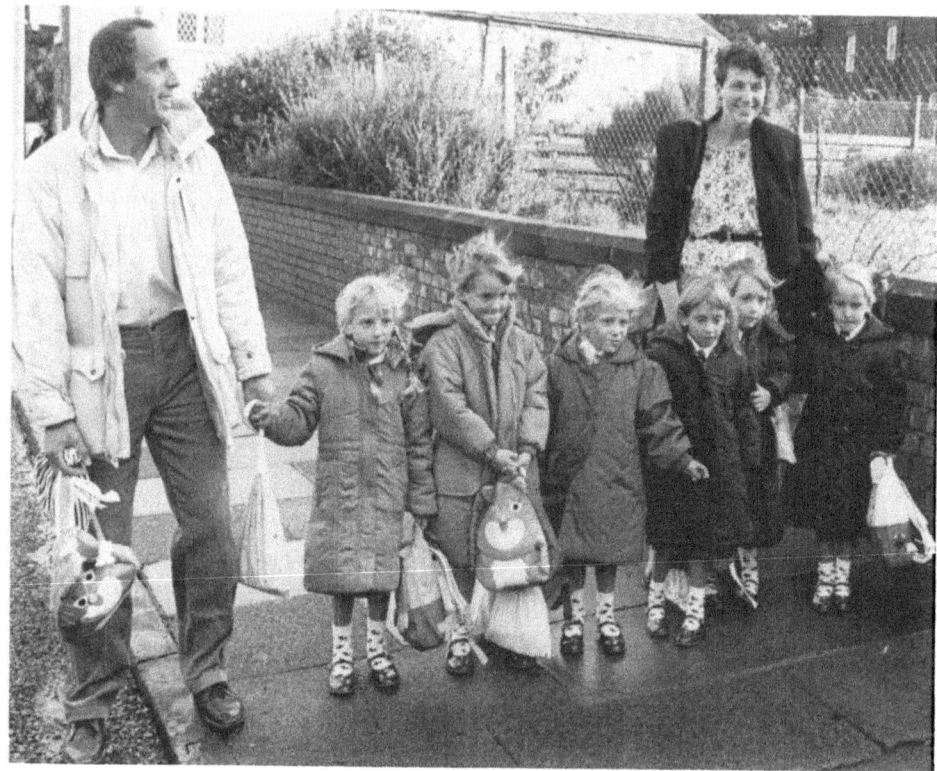

Fig. 2.2. The Walton sextuplets face the cameras after their first day at school. The *Guardian* (13 September 1988) reported: 'Their parents, Graham and Janet Walton, took the six, who will be five on November 18, to school at St George's Primary, in Wallasey, the Wirral, Merseyside. After assembly, the six . . . were paired into three groups: Hannah and Jenny in one class, Kate and Ruth in another, and Lucy and Sarah in a third. The headmaster, The Reverend Bruce Harry, said they were split up because "if they had all gone into one reception class the teacher would have found difficulty balancing the time she gave them and the other children. This will let them develop at their own pace. There were no tears. They are settled in very happily."' (Photo: Mercury Press Agency.)

higher average birthweight than is usual (the 1990 *Guinness Book of Records** gives their total weight as 10,915g).

A further live sextuplet delivery occurred in January 1980 in Florence, Italy (Giavanaucci *et al.* 1981). By careful prenatal management, gestation was brought to 34.5 weeks and the babies, four boys and two girls, were all in good health, weighing from 1200 to 1750g. In a follow-up report at 2 years, Levi d'Ancona *et al.* (1982) stated that 'they all seem faring very well with no neurological or psychological deficit.'

Of the six sets of sextuplets born in England and Wales since 1952 (see Table 2.I, p. 16), two sets have survived intact: the Waltons (Fig. 2.2) and the Colemans (Fig. 2.3).

*The *Guinness Book of Records* is ©1989, Guinness Publishing Ltd., Enfield, Middlesex.

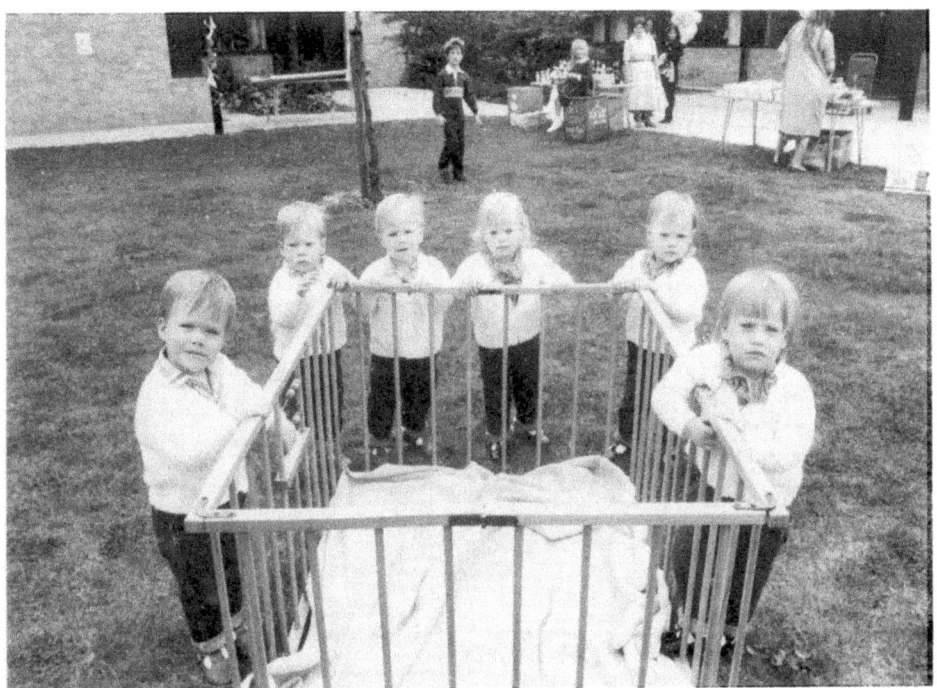

Fig. 2.3. The Coleman sextuplets lend 'a dozen helping hands' (*Sunday Times*, 18 September 1988) to the launch of a national campaign for special baby care units, held at the Homerton Hospital, London, where they were born two years previously. (Photo: Times Newspapers Ltd.)

In addition to the above cases, because of fetal damage, stillbirths or postnatal death on the one hand and selective abortion (Serreyn *et al.* 1984, Duchatel and Mennesson 1985, Price 1988) on the other, members of several living multiple sets derive from higher gestations.*

Quintuplets have been reported in larger numbers and a full review is not possible here. One notable early example was recorded in a illustrated 'broadside' of 1566, reproduced overleaf (Fig. 2.4). A history of the scientific study of quins might begin with the set reported by Garthshore in 1787. Margaret Waddington, 'a poor woman of the township of Lower Darwin, near Blackburn in Lancashire', gave birth on 25 April 1786 to five girls, two live and three stillborn.

Each child presented naturally, was preceded by a separate burst of water, and was delivered by the natural pains only. In a short time after the birth of the last, the placenta was expelled by nature without any haemorrhage, was uncommonly large, and in some places beginning to be putrid. It consisted of one uniform continued cake, and was not divided into distinct placentulae, the lobulated appearance being nearly equal all over. Each funis was contained

---

*The Dionne quins may in fact have originated as sextuplets. Dafoe (1934) reported that the mother 'gave a history of labor-like pains for two hours at the beginning of the third month, after which she passed from the vagina a black oval object about the size of a duck's egg, streaked with white and firm in consistency.' However, this was not preserved and therefore 'no conclusion as to the possibility of another pregnancy could be made.'

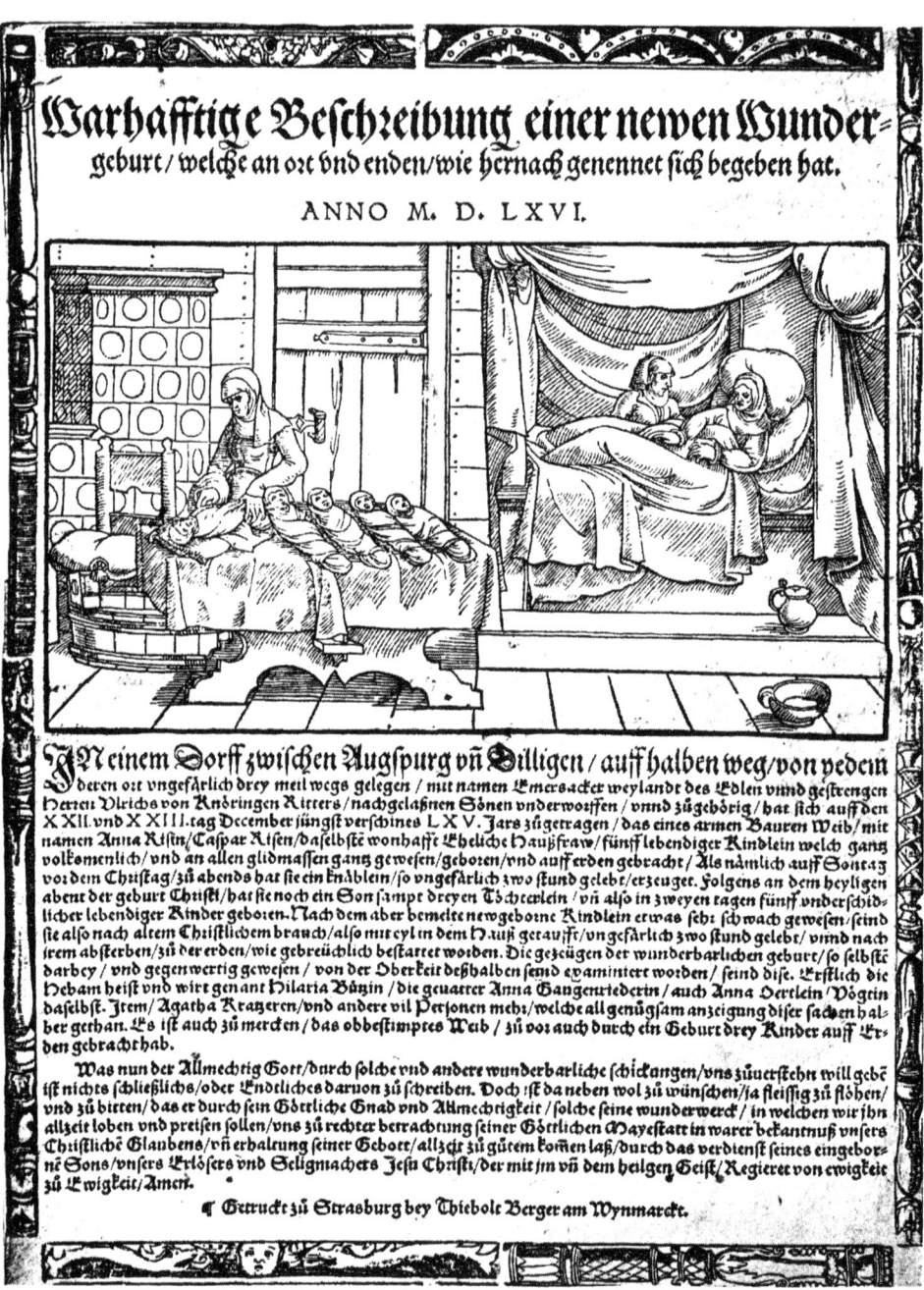

Fig. 2.4. Illustrated 'broadside' of 1566, reproduced from an article by McDaniels (1942) in which the German text is translated in part as follows: 'In a village situated half-way between Augsburg and Dillingen, about three miles from each, Emersacker by name . . . it came about that on the 22d and 23d day of December of the 65th year just passed, Anna, the wife of a poor peasant, Caspar Risen, dwelling in that place, a married housewife, gave birth to and was delivered of five living infants who were entirely complete and possessed of all the members. Namely, on the Sunday before Christmas, in the

in a separate cell, within which each child had been lodged; and it was easy to perceive, by the state of the funis, and that part of the placenta to which it adhered, in which sac the dead, and in which the living children had been contained. I examined the septa of the cells very carefully, but could not divide them as usual into distinct laminae, nor determine which was chorion or which amnios. I could not prevail on the good women to allow me to carry it home, to be more narrowly inspected; and I submitted more readily to their prejudice for its being burned, as its very soft texture seemed to me to render it hardly capable to bear injection. The two living children having survived their birth but a short time, I was allowed to carry them home; and I have preserved the whole five in spirits.

The dead infants, thus preserved, were exhibited to the Royal Society of Medicine in 1787 and subsequently deposited in the museum of the Royal College of Surgeons. During the Second World War, as a precaution against air raid damage, such specimens were removed to the University of Toronto, where Norma Ford Walker had earlier studied the footprints of the Dionne quins as a possible means of determining their zygosity (MacArthur and Ford 1937). In a subsequent investigation (Walker 1950) she found the 1786 babies to be so beautifully preserved that it was possible—more than 160 years later—to take their footprints and establish with some confidence that they were an MZ set!

From that time until the birth of the Dionnes there are no reports of survivors from a quintuplet conception, although it is always possible that one or two babies did survive from such a set but that the event was not thought worthy of report. The Dionnes' survival, and the fact that they were an MZ set, was partly responsible for the attention they attracted.

Nine years later the next quintuplet set to survive, the Diligentis, were born in Argentina (Beruti 1944); they were reared away from the glare of publicity as the family deliberately sought to avoid the attention that had surrounded the Dionnes. By 1954 Nichols was able to publish an account of 14 verified quintuplet births in the USA and Canada between 1826 and 1950, but of these the Dionnes were the only survivors. There are now many reports of surviving quintuplet sets—from England, Poland, Israel, Japan, South Africa and New Zealand—most proceeding through childhood with normal development. The earliest fertility drug sets have now reached adulthood. With the exception of the 'Danzig quins' (see Chapter 5, pp. 53–55), no quintuplet set has been studied developmentally in a systematic way for an extensive period.

The rise and fall of psychology's interest
The period of high interest
To understand the active interest of psychologists—especially in North America—in higher order births in the years from 1929 to 1944, it is necessary to turn to a history of three movements—the maternal and infant health movement, the child development movement, and the interest in twins for the scientific study of genetics and human development.

---

evening, she produced a little boy, who lived about two hours. Subsequently, on the holy eve of Christ's birth she gave birth to another son together with three little daughters, and thus, in two days, to five separate living children. But inasmuch as the aforesaid new-born children were very feeble, they were hastily baptized in the house, following the Christian custom, and lived about two hours. After their death they were buried in the ground, as is usual.'

THE MATERNAL AND INFANT WELFARE MOVEMENT

Concern for infant welfare in France, Britain and other European countries arose from a fear of depopulation in the late 19th century when infant mortality was exceptionally high and the major killers were gastroenteritis, respiratory and other infectious diseases. Proper infant care, suitable feeding and methods of nursing were identified as areas for attention, and training courses for midwives, registration of midwives and the establishment of milk banks to support infant feeding programmes all date from the early 1900s. At one level this concern arose from consideration for persons at risk, but at another level it fitted with political and ideological recognition that increasing prosperity depended on an increasing population who would inherit the earth. Information became available through the maternal and child health movement that would be related in some way to the survival of more multiple sets after the first decade of this century.

THE CHILD DEVELOPMENT MOVEMENT

Gesell's Yale Clinic for Child Development began in 1911, and in 1930 Robert Woodward founded the Society for Research in Child Development. Between these two dates the child study movement in the USA emerged (Senn 1975), and by 1935 Woodward had launched an impressive publications programme for the Society.

During the 1920s, to meet the need for systematic knowledge about child development, around 10 child study institutes were created through the zeal of Lawrence Frank and with the support of the Laura Spelman Rockefeller funds. For a quarter of a century the field could be defined almost entirely in terms of a few places—Iowa, Minnesota, Berkeley, Antioch, Yale, Toronto, Detroit, Columbia—and the people located there. The child study institutes were accumulating longitudinal and cross-sectional normative data on growth and child behaviours.

There was a demand for better scientific methodologies and for tools appropriate to the study of children (Anderson, *in* Senn 1975). Questions were asked about theoretical formulations which might guide the study of babies from birth through the early years: what records and observations could be made? The interests of the child study research institutes in the USA were strongly reinforced by the active preschool movement in the 1920s and by the progressive education movement in that country.

Contemporaneously, psychology's interest in children of higher multiple birth began to gather momentum. It is within this historical context that scientific interest in the first widely reported sets must be seen: the Keys quadruplets (born 1916, reported 1931); the first surviving MZ quadruplets, the Morloks (born 1930); and the first surviving quintuplets, the Dionnes (born 1934).

TWIN STUDIES

In the early 1930s there was still doubt as to whether two different kinds of twins existed. As a result of Galton's work and advocacy of the contribution that twin studies could make to questions of heredity (*e.g.* Galton 1875), psychologists saw a role not just in using twins for psychological research but also in solving the questions of zygosity.

Both in the child study institutes of the USA and in the laboratories of the Soviet Union twin studies were exploring the genetic control of simple and complex motor learning (Hilgard 1933, Mirenva 1935). Although one might argue for the quality of these studies in most respects, researchers had to base the establishment of zygosity on questionable indices of similarity. There was a more general interest in questions concerning child development, such as 'What is an optimum environment?' or 'What benefits can come from particular treatment of children during their growing years?' Terman's study of gifted children (Terman 1925, 1954) was already under way at this time, as was a large longitudinal study at Berkeley (see Senn 1975).

The first psychological study of a quadruplet set to be published appeared in 1931. This was Brintle's comprehensive case study of the Keys quadruplets at 12 years. On physical growth and psychological variables the zygosity groupings appeared obvious: they must be an MZ and a DZ pair.

In a report on an MZ set of girl quadruplets (the Morloks), Clarke (1932) argued for the particular advantages of a study of children each with the same set of genes. Gardner and Newman (1943b) studied the same set later in childhood, and predicted that in years to come such children might teach us much regarding the connections between heredity and environment.

A PIVOTAL EVENT

Several more live births of quadruplets were reported between 1930 and 1935 but received only minor attention. In 1934 the Dionnes survived a fiction-like birth (see p. 28) to become the first living set of quintuplets (Dafoe 1934, 1936, 1940; Dafoe and Dafoe 1937) (Fig. 2.5). They were also diagnosed to be an MZ set. This brought to one point of focus much of the earlier scientific interest. Two acts of chance caused them to hold that focus for many decades. Their doctor's brother held a position in the medical school of the University of Toronto where an Institute of Child Study had been established for psychological research. Through this contact other professional resources became available for the guiding and recording of the Dionnes' progress, and reports found publication outlets. The second act of fate was that, when the next surviving set of quintuplets (the Diligentis) were born nine years later, the parents shunned all publicity, and it was the mid-1960s before other quintuplet births received much popular attention. Early scientific interest in the Dionnes centred upon their zygosity, and how one zygote could divide to create five babies. The interest of the child study movement was reflected in questions like 'How should they be treated?', 'How would they grow up?', 'Would they be normal?' and 'How similar or different would they become as older children or as adults?'

When the Dionne quins were 10 months old Dr W. E. Blatz, Professor of Child Psychology at the University of Toronto and Director of the Institute of Child Study, began to observe their mental and emotional growth and to supervise their preschool education. By this action their medical advisers gave early recognition to the importance of psychological development. By the mid-1930s the psychological study of child development and its relationship to child-rearing practices and nursery school education was fairly advanced and this was a legitimate area for research. Careful records were kept of their progress up to the age of 4 years (Blatz 1937, 1939) (Fig. 2.6).

Professional interest in the Dionnes was sufficiently widespread for a conference to be called to report on the early studies. Many wished to attend; only some could be accommodated. Child psychologists were among the scientists present. Several of these studies were collated into a single volume (Blatz et al. 1937), now long out of print (although I was advised by the University of Toronto Press that it may soon be available again in some reproduced form). Newman's comment on the quins captures the meaning of the event for scientists at that time:

> The real importance of the quins is that they represent a highly scientific experiment performed by nature; an experiment so rare that it behoves us to make the most of it by trying to understand it as fully as possible and by drawing from it as much new knowledge as our powers of observation and deduction will permit. (Newman 1942)

The decline of interest

Ten years after the birth of the Dionnes interest in multiple children, their growth and development dropped, and documentation almost disappeared from the psychological literature. It reappeared in a specialist form in the 1950s in a new journal for twin studies edited by Luigi Gedda (the *Acta Geneticae Medicae et Gemellologiae*). A possible contributory factor to this decline was the historical shift in emphasis of the methods to be used in psychological research.

Robinson and Foster (1979) described the rise and fall of studies involving small numbers of children ('small-N studies') in three phases:

> From 1870 to 1920 small-N studies relied on constancy and elimination as control for secondary variables.
>
> From 1920 to 1970 experimental approaches included a large number of subjects using randomization, statistical control, independent variables, control groups and statistical analyses of the findings.
>
> From 1960 there has been a rise in publication of studies using a small number of subjects, the cultivation of elimination and constancy as control techniques, repeated measures taken from each subject, a control condition allowing for self-contained means of determining significance of results and typically no statistical analysis of data.

In methodological texts headings appear like 'A Return to the Individual' (Hersen and Barlow 1976). The term 'case study research' has taken on new meanings in time series studies where the unit can consist of a single subject, a group or a social system, and measurement involves the unit measured repeatedly or the unit replicated (Kratochwill 1978). (The reader will begin to sense a rationale for a revived interest in the use of repeated measures on the individuals in a multiple set.)

By the 1920s studies of large populations using Fischer's approach to data analysis were well-established in the psychological literature and, one suspects, in publication policies. The headings 'Quadruplets' and 'Quintuplets' disappeared from *Psychological Abstracts* after 1960. Professional credit would not accrue to the researcher engaged in small-N studies of multiple sets of children, support from colleagues could be absent and editorial policies might block publication.

There was no lack of subjects in the 1945–1965 period. New multiple sets were born and survived. In subtle ways the worldwide publicity given to the Dionnes had adverse effects on public opinion concerning children of multiple sets, on the attitudes of parents and even on professional interest. The suspicion that children in multiple sets were abnormal, were treated abnormally by their environments, or would become abnormal as a result of their multiple status increased and could not be dispelled because no data were gathered. In the 1950s psychiatric illness was diagnosed in a set of quadruplets (Rosenthal 1963). Then Emilie Dionne's epilepsy became public knowledge with her death in 1954 and later Marie Dionne's death was interpreted by the media to be the result of depression and mental ill-health. Berton's book, *The Dionne Years: A Thirties Melodrama* (1977), is the most recent contributor to this cloud of atypicality that has surrounded children in multiple sets. Against this one could set the history of the Gehris (*b*.1880), the high-achieving Keys quads (*b*.1915), the Johnsons (*b*.1935), the Goods (otherwise known as the 'Bristol quads'—*b*.1948), the Wroclaw quads (*b*.1954) and many other normally developing sets, although other sets have included one or more members with a mental or physical impairment.

This sense of atypicality is not only held by the public and fed by the media: researchers and other professionals also have contributed their opinions to it. When objective accounts of the growth and development of higher multiple groups appear in greater number, then perhaps this cloud will be dispersed.

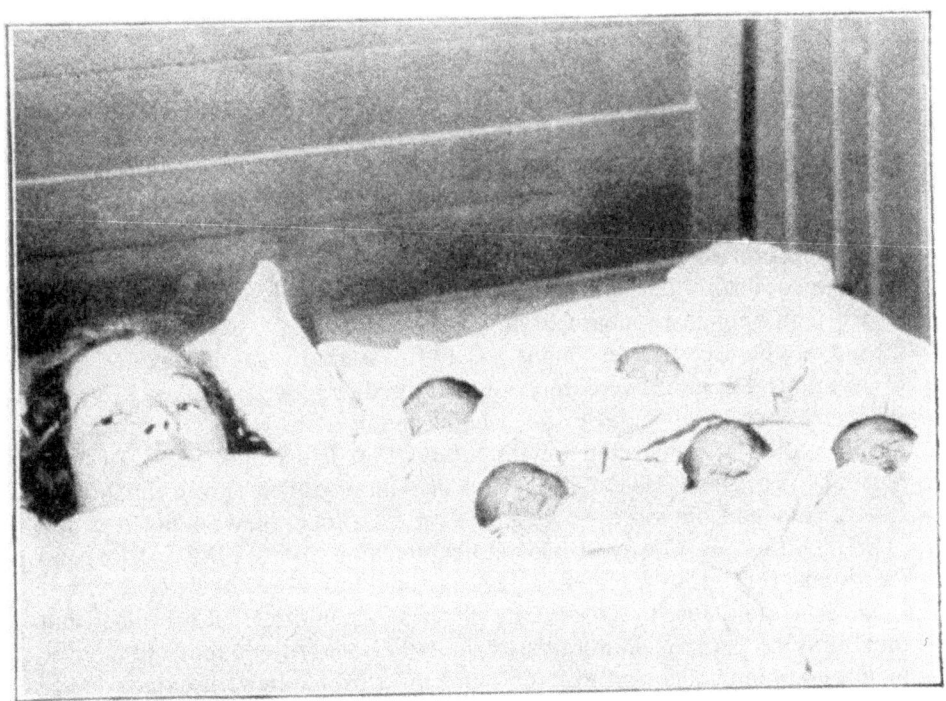

Fig. 2.5. Mrs. Elzire Dionne with her five babies, aged 2 days (Dafoe 1934).

FAIRY TALES AND SCIENTIFIC ENQUIRIES

The British Medical Journal (1934) described the birth of the Dionne quintuplets as an 'astonishing event' and an 'incredible affair', and in a subsequent report the attending doctor referred to it as a 'medical fairy tale'.

When he was called to the Dionne cottage at 4am on May 28th, 1934, Dr Dafoe had expected to deliver a single baby. However . .

> I arrived to find the home in confusion, no preparation made for confinement, except a tea-kettle boiling on the stove. Two babies had already been born, and a third was just making its appearance over the perineum. Two neighbors were acting as midwives. The father had disappeared. I scrubbed up in the best way available, took over the situation, and delivered the third baby. The neighbors then scurried about the house to get some wrappings for the babies and replenish the fire. In the meantime another amniotic sac was presenting itself at the vaginal orifice and a little pressure over the abdomen brought another baby into the world. This was followed by still another.
>
> In the early hours of the morning and still sleepy from a previous obstetric case that night, the whole situation seemed to be unreal and dreamlike, but I mechanically went about the business of looking after the babies . . . I didn't see how all of the babies could possibly live, so I baptized them separately. They were then wrapped in the only covering available, which proved to be remnants of cotton sheeting and old napkins, and then laid on the corner of the bed and covered with a heated blanket.
>
> The mother in the meantime was not recovering and my attention was immediately called to her condition. Blood was oozing away and . . . she presented the appearance of a dying woman. The husband was still missing and it was my duty to get the priest, as no one else was available with a car. (Dafoe 1934)

Upon his return he found the mother and children all alive, but the placenta carried away and destroyed: this was a loss to science, as membrane analysis was crucial at that time for determining zygosity. There is a possible discrepancy between Dafoe's report that the last two babies 'were born within intact amniotic sacs and could be seen moving their arms and legs through the transparent walls' and a later comment by Norma Ford Walker to Scheinfeld (1968) that the midwives floated out the membrane in a tub of water and that there were probably only two amniotic sacs and a single chorion. No record was made of birth order, and no birthweights were recorded as there were no scales small enough to measure the separate weights of the babies. On the second day their combined weight was 13 lbs. 6 oz. (about 6065g).

Various attempts were made to study the genetic similarity of the children. They were found to have many features in common. Similarities were reported of height and weight (MacArthur and Dafoe 1939), of taste reactions (Ford and Mason 1941) and of dental growth (Ford and Mason 1943). They had the same webbed toes on each foot; they belonged to the same blood group (O); eyes, hair and complexion differed little; palm- and footprints were closely matched (MacArthur and Ford 1937, MacArthur 1938, Scheinfeld 1968). Considering all these similarities, and the fact that there was no history of multiparity in either parent's immediate family, medical opinion concurred that the quins most probably were monozygotic.

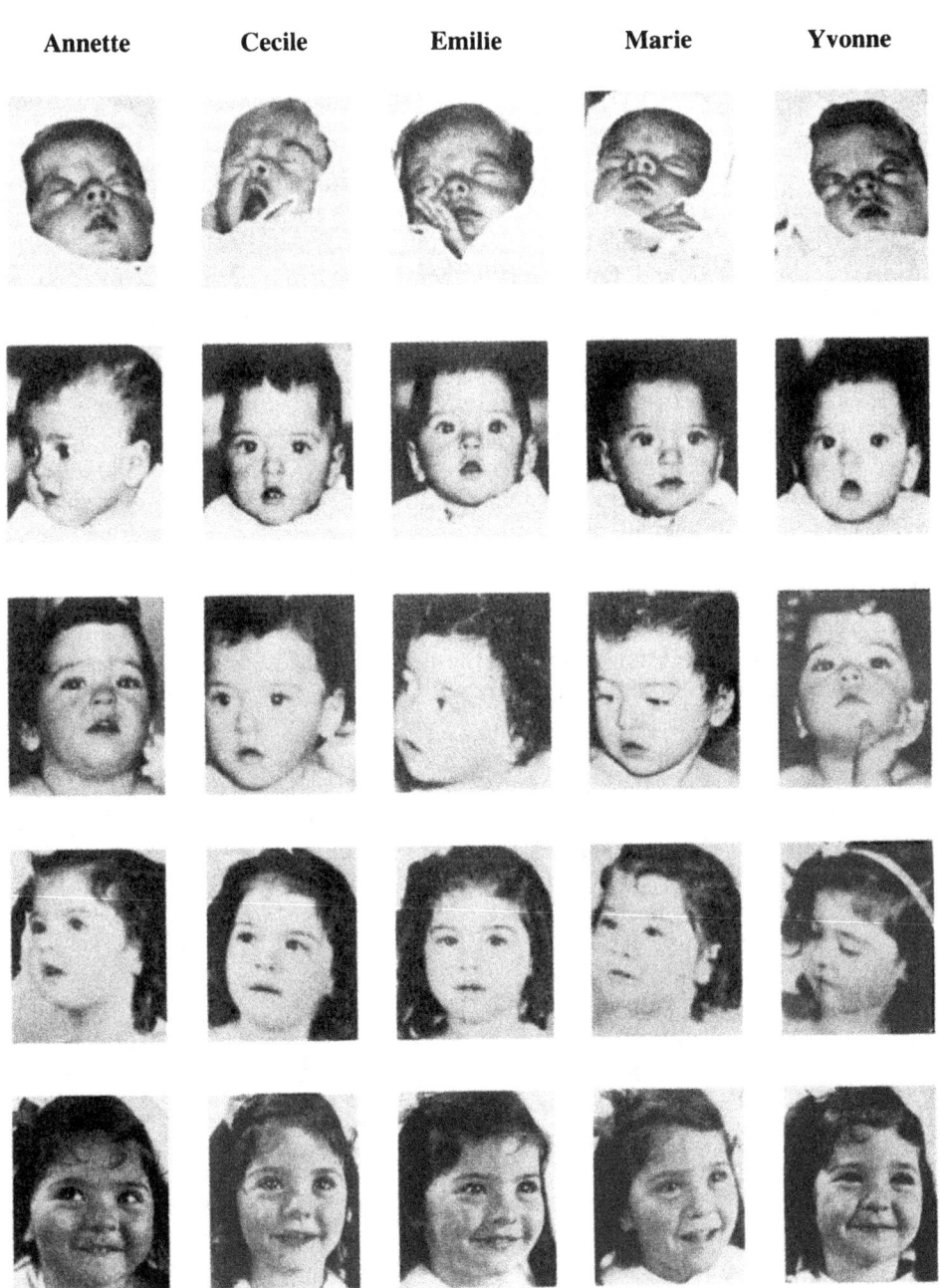

Fig. 2.6. The Dionne quintuplets, photographed at 3, 9, 18, 40 and 48 months (Blatz 1939).

3
PREGNANCY AND BIRTH

The diagnosis of multiple pregnancy
In historical cases of multiple pregnancy it was the mother's rapid increase in size that was seen as exceptional and this would give rise to further checks. Often a mother would go close to full term or even into labour before a multiple birth was suspected (Shepherd and Potter 1949). Most modern reports indicate that at around five months suspicions have been checked, either by X-ray or, more recently, by ultrasonography. In most cases where ultrasonography is not available, multiple pregnancy is signalled by the mother's symptoms which are unlike those in singleton pregnancies of the same duration.

In vitro fertilization has introduced many new factors into the multiple birth area, and one related to diagnosis was reported by Kanhai *et al.* (1986). A 34-year-old mother whose first pregnancy had been induced by hormone therapy was found to be pregnant again after a second treatment and at five weeks ultrasonography revealed a quintuplet pregnancy. This caused considerable distress and was unacceptable to the couple, who requested termination. Full discussion led to a successful attempt to reduce the number of fetuses from quins to twins at 10 weeks. After an uneventful pregnancy the mother went into spontaneous labour and gave birth to two healthy daughters with birthweights of 2620g and 2360g.

Management of the prenatal period
Multiple pregnancy is a very important obstetric and paediatric problem because of the very high perinatal mortality rates (Green 1967). There is a challenge to get the mother as far along her pregnancy as possible (McFee *et al.* 1974) and to delay the onset of preterm labour. Doctors are concerned on the one hand with the mother's resources to continue with the pregnancy and on the other with the development of the fetuses to as mature a state as possible before birth. The average length of gestation varies inversely with the number of fetuses. According to a review by McKeown and Record (1952), most quadruplets were delivered between 32 and 36 weeks, many were delivered before that and only one went to 38 weeks.

Stewart (1982) noted that several surveys conducted over the previous decade had shown little change in the rate of undiagnosed multiple births, which had remained at around 23 per cent. It was argued that the disadvantages of an undiagnosed multiple birth lie in the medical, emotional, financial and environmental effects on the parents and their babies, and on the family unit particularly when other siblings are involved. The appeal was for more attention to early diagnosis.

Prenatal risk factors
Any study of a higher multiple birth must take into account that their survival as a complete set may have been due to certain favourable prenatal conditions. Thus all

sources of information about the prenatal period, the confinement and the time during which the medical team remained in contact with the family are important and records should be kept. Position, crowding and conditions of delivery, for instance, are environmental factors which are peculiar to multiple births and tend to affect the last two months of growth.

MZ conceptions, which occur less often than DZ conceptions, are subject to particular risks. They are more likely to suffer malformations. Those who develop in a single chorion with one amniotic sac (the most delayed type of duplication; see Fig. 3.1) are especially vulnerable, and they are more likely to have some disruption to the prenatal supply of nutrients, as connections which develop in the blood vessels of a common placenta may favour one fetus over another, and these may operate from a very early stage of gestation (Schatz 1882, Myrianthopoulos 1975). Schinzel et al. (1979) made a study of structural defects in a large sample of MZ twins and concluded that the aetiology of twinning is a cause of early morphogenesis in one or both fetuses, especially in the single chorion, single amnion type. They recommended that, to determine zygosity, a careful examination should be made of the birth membranes and placenta, and when there is a malformed fetus they should also be checked for evidence of a deceased or incomplete twin.

Prenatal factors, then, can cause physical differences between MZ fetuses which began life genetically matched. These would include:
★ malformations caused by the same agents that cause late duplications (which can be concordant in both twins or nonconcordant affecting only one twin);
★ overcrowding in the uterus, affecting the fetuses either directly or indirectly;
★ connections between blood vessels which disrupt the supply of nutrients (Bhargava et al. 1971);
★ the remote possibility of somatic mutation.

The birth
McFee et al. (1974) listed the birth problems associated with higher multiple gestations as: uterine inertia; difficulties in the second stage of labour (fetal malposition, haemorrhage from the placental separation or cord prolapse); and postpartum haemorrhage. Each of these problems could occur in a singleton birth; in a multiple birth each successive fetus may be more at risk. Plans for the arrival of four or more babies must be made in several areas—preparedness is an essential element in the care of the babies (Dunkley 1967, Spillman 1987). Keast and Cooper (1967) listed: an early planning meeting of obstetric, paediatric, anaesthetic and nursing staff; preparations for the confinement; and preparations for the immediate and continuing paediatric care of the children. In a report of two concurrent quadruplet pregnancies managed at the John Radcliffe Hospital in Oxford, Salisbury et al. (1977) stressed the need for adequate staffing and neonatal equipment, especially in the case of preterm, low-birthweight multiple deliveries (see pp. 157–158). Most recent reports have included brief notes on the management of the birth in hospital—VaFai and Shapiro (1985) discussed this in some detail. Aherne (1983) reported an interesting account of a quadruplet delivery in Tanzania with limited resources (see p. 162).

Most reported cases had a short first stage of labour, probably related to the small size of each baby and to the fact that the mothers had had two or more babies previously. Problems at the second stage of labour relate to the positions of the babies at presentation. If they are under 32 weeks' gestation there is little trouble, but for those 32 weeks and over the greater size of the babies may cause positioning and 'queueing' problems. A difficult and prolonged delivery of one fetus may adversely affect those that follow. Caesarian section is increasingly preferred in such cases, especially if a rapid delivery is indicated on medical grounds. It can be carried out by arrangement, and it can result in a very short birth period with a minimum time between the delivery of each baby. In one such birth, reported by Hamilton et al. (1959), the four babies were delivered in less than two minutes, the operation proceeding uneventfully and taking in all 25 minutes. More children have been surviving multiple birth in the last two decades and the loss of some or all of the babies is often averted by careful preparations and good teamwork.

Rates of caesarian delivery are much higher for multiples of all categories than for singleton births. In one American report, Placek et al. (1983) found that the overall rate of caesarian births had increased from 4.5 per cent in 1965 to 17.9 per cent in 1981, and that the rates were higher for low-birthweight babies. For multiple births the frequency rose to 24.4 per cent.

Except for the mother who has already had twins or triplets, the birth experience will be a strange and novel one. From their reports of higher multiple deliveries I gained the impression that many co-operative mothers had worked well with their doctors to bring their babies into the world. Some had requested analgesics or anaesthesia, others wanted only minimum pain relief.

Determination of zygosity

Questions of zygosity were rarely conclusively established from the time children of higher multiple births began to survive until the 1960s, although physical characteristics and dermatoglyphics were carefully compared in the more highly researched sets. Despite the difficulties often surrounding these births, the importance of establishing zygosity by placental or membrane examination and of securing blood and/or placental tissue samples at the time must be re-emphasized.

Information on zygosity in multiple births is of importance not only for epidemiological, genetic and obstetrical studies but also because of the difference in prognosis between MZ and DZ sets. Furthermore, the parents themselves usually want to know, not least because their chances of having multiple births in future pregnancies will vary according to the zygosity. Nevertheless it is unfortunately still relatively uncommon for the zygosity to be determined at birth. After that time valuable information from the placenta will have been lost and blood samples become harder to collect.

Methods
SEX
Within a set clearly those of different sex cannot be monozygotic (with the extremely rare exception of a case of heterokaryotopic chromosomal anomaly where a normal XY male has an XO female MZ twin (Riekhof et al. 1972).

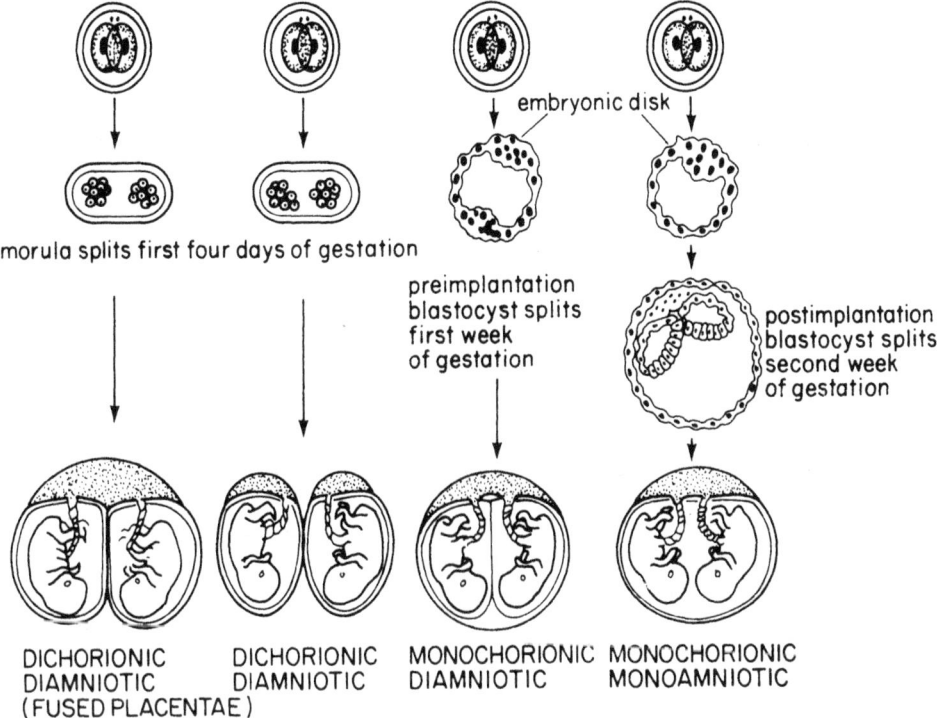

Fig. 3.1. Different possibilities for development and plancentation in monozygotic twins (Fox 1978).

PLACENTATION

In multiple births the number of chorionic sacs* must be established. A monochorionic placenta is proof of monozygosity. However, the converse is *not* true. In the one-third of MZ cases where division occurs within the first three days or so after fertilization, the fetuses will have separate chorions. The dichorionic placenta is then anatomically indistinguishable from that of a DZ fetus and the placental discs may remain separate or may fuse together depending on the site of implantation (Strong and Corney 1967). The different forms of placentation in MZ twins are illustrated in Figure 3.1.

Accurate descriptions of placentae in higher multiple births tend to be limited to case reports. Little attention has been given to the frequency of the various chorion types as in most studies the numbers are too small. On the same pattern as for twins, the placentae of all TZ triplets will be trichorionic, and one-third of DZ triplets should also have three chorions, whereas two-thirds will be dichorionic. On the same grounds one-ninth of MZ triplets should be trichorionic, four-ninths dichorionic and four-ninths monochorionic. The frequency of the different types of placentation in higher order births can be estimated in the same way.

*The *chorion* is the outer membrane surrounding the fetus; the *annion* is the inner membrane.

In like-sex children with dichorionic placentae other methods of zygosity determination must be used.

PHYSICAL FEATURES

In older children and adults physical features are a relatively good means of establishing zygosity (Cohen *et al.* 1975, Kasriel and Eaves 1976). But appearances are of little help in newborn twins, on whom intrauterine influences may well be stronger than genetic ones, particularly in cases of the fetofetal transfusion syndrome when MZ twins may have large intrapair weight discrepancies (Bryan 1983).

BLOOD GROUPING

The most useful genetically determined characteristics to study are those, like blood groups, with a simple mode of inheritance and commonly occurring variations. Tests are most practicably done on cord blood samples but can of course be carried out at any age. More recently other genetic markers such as red cell enzymes, serum proteins, and tissue enzymes (in particular from the placenta) have been used. If any marker differs, the infants cannot be MZ. Monozygosity cannot be proven by marker testing, but the probability increases with the number of markers tested and the exact mathematical probability can be calculated (this will be more precise if the parents' race and blood types are known) (Corney and Robson 1975).

DNA PROBES

A new and highly reliable tool for testing zygosity is the minisatellite DNA probe which detects many regions of great variability on the human genome and provides a much greater degree of accuracy than any previous test (Derom *et al.* 1985, Hill and Jeffreys 1985). An added advantage is that only small volumes of blood (or placental tissue) are needed.

4
FAMILY CONTEXT AND RELATIONSHIPS

The crisis of multiple pregnancy and birth
Caplan (1961) explored the nature of crises and possible helpful interventions. A crisis is provoked when a person faces an obstacle to important life goals which, for a time, is insurmountable using customary methods of problem solving. A period of disorganization ensues, a period of upset, during which many different abortive attempts at solution are made. Eventually some kind of adaptation is achieved.

By Caplan's description the whole course of pregnancy might be considered a time of crisis because 'it is a period of altered behaviour; it is a period of disequilibrium compared with the normal state of family life; it is a period of emotional upset in the woman and often in her husband and her other children; and it is a period when there are problems, many of which cannot adequately be handled by use of the normal problem solving mechanisms.'

However, a pregnancy of 30–40 weeks is rather too long to be conceptualized as a crisis: it is a period which may be seen to have a stable life of its own. It is a time during which the number of hazardous circumstances is likely to increase, the potential for feeling a sense of threat or loss is higher, the obstacles to reaching one's life goals may increase, and it is harder to use one's past repertoire of problem solving methods. With such sensitivities the mother may revive old fears, fantasies and ideas.

Rose (1961) compiled a series of contingencies that seem, singly or in combination, to be critical stresses associated with mothering breakdown and potential sources of pathogenic mother–infant interaction. From his list of 14 factors, those which are particularly relevant to the study of quads and higher multiple sets would be:
★ multiple birth itself;
★ previous abortions, periods of sterility, traumatic past deliveries, loss of previous children;
★ health complications during pregnancy;
★ moving away from the family group or back to the group at a critical period for mother and child (for bed-rest in hospital, for example);
★ dislocating moves in pregnancy or the neonatal period involving changing geographical area and the need to find new ties;
★ children born within 10 or 12 months of each other.

Other authors have demonstrated the mental health hazards for mothers of preterm babies. Cadden (1962) suggested that while there may be some warning of preterm delivery in multiple birth there are liable to be many features similar to preterm singleton births—an atmosphere of emergency; an air of apprehensiveness; unbelievably small babies, perhaps frighteningly unattractive in appearance. There may be real dangers that the babies will not live, or may not be normal. They may need intensive care and be separated from the mother, and in some cases may stay in hospital long after the mother has gone home. It is possible to summarize in a general way the kind of help that a person in crisis needs, but each birth of a higher multiple set will be accompanied by a special set of circumstances.

Most mothers have some fears during pregnancy that there will be damage to themselves or to their babies.

Many obstetricians will say that one of the first questions a mother asks after delivery is "Is the baby all right?" And one of the first things many wise obstetricians do is to show the mother the baby and to tell her, "He has all his fingers and toes." (Caplan 1961)

Such concerns about abnormality are not so easily allayed in the case of higher multiple births; more of such infants are stillborn or abnormal. Everyone around the mother could be telling her something different because so little is known about this rare occurrence.

Only the more recent medical reports comment on the mental health of mothers at this time. Most of these mothers already have children, and a long period of hospitalization means an unwanted separation for mother, children and husband. If the expectant mother facing a singleton birth has some uncertainties before her, the mother awaiting the birth of a large group of children faces many more. Some of the negative answers carry quite high probabilities. How many children will there be? How will she manage the birth? Will the babies be healthy and normal? Will they all survive? Does she really want that many children? How will she manage with them at home? How will the family afford the necessities for so many children? Even the long periods of hospitalization can have their consequences and McFee *et al.* (1974) list neuroses from bed-rest as one of the problems of the neonatal period. There is little literature the mother can turn to for information (*e.g.* see Catalogue entry on Crawley quads, p. 166). When she has read the books on the Dionnes and a few magazine articles she is on her own in unmapped territory as far as her friends, relatives and community are concerned, and she is very dependent on the guidance of her medical advisers. (Support groups have been established in some countries in recent years—see Appendix 2.)

Burnell (1974) reported the obstetric history of a septuplet pregnancy from which none of the children survived, and the psychiatric history of that mother's adjustment and how she managed her next pregnancy. He concluded that the experience of multiple birth is a stressful event because of the following considerations:

(1) There is an element of unknown and unexpected occurrence. (2) The event is rare, and attracts immediate attention and publicity. (3) The prematurity raises anxiety about possible complications and loss of life. There may be grief about a partial or total loss. (4) The event may bring on feelings of inadequacy, ambivalence, or guilt in certain predisposed individuals. (5) The reactions of the spouse, grandparents, and friends can be either supportive or further stress-producing.

In the case reported by Burnell the mother made a satisfactory physical and psychological recovery and adjustment. Factors contributing to this according to Burnell were:

(1) The patient was given the privacy needed for her to go through the expected grief and the need to have some time alone. (2) She was offered the opportunity to talk about her

grief, her feelings of inadequacy and her future goals with a psychiatrist. (3) She was shielded from the pressures for publicity in the press and television. (4) Her spouse remained supportive, protective, and hopeful of the future. (5) She received much support from her obstetrician, in whom she had complete trust. (6) The nursing staff was protective and very responsive to all of her needs.

The psychiatric intervention has several functions in such cases. It is to prevent unresolved guilt or grief; to facilitate the grief reaction by giving the patient an opportunity to review the meaning of the loss in her own life experience; and to make appropriate recommendations for psychosocial support for the mother, and to provide support and guidance to the father and other relatives if necessary. It is only possible here to summarize the ways in which to assist a mother in crisis:
★ help her confront the crisis;
★ help her confront the crisis in manageable doses;
★ help her to find the facts;
★ do not give false assurances;
★ do not encourage her to blame others;
★ help her to accept help;
★ help her with everyday tasks.

Caplan's writings explore and explain these strategies further.

Services provided for the family

The families of the first surviving sets of quads or quins (Dionnes, Morloks, Diligentis) were not faced with hospital expenses. Today, however, as more special care is prescribed for the mother and her babies, the birth can prove very expensive in those countries which do not have a free health service.

Reports of quads born in the 1930s describe the financial hardships, the space problems and the child care demands placed on the parents of higher multiple sets.

The Morlok quadruplets suffered the same prenatal, natal and early postnatal handicaps as did the Dionne quintuplets and their survival as a group of vigorous, healthy and intelligent youngsters is only a little less remarkable than that of the quints. They had, moreover, no personal physician, no trained personal nurses or governesses whose sole duty it was to look after their health and education. No commodious home was especially designed and built for them, and no special police guarded them day and night. Because they were born almost four years before scientific and popular interest in human multiple births had been aroused by the dramatic advent of the quintuplets, the birth of these quadruplets was only moderately publicized. They were given very little help by the community. At the time of their birth Mr Morlok was unemployed. He was helped by the city of Lansing to the extent of being given a modest dwelling, rent free. He was subsequently appointed city constable, a position he still holds. (Gardner and Newman 1943*b*)

The father of the [Schense] quadruplets was a farmer of German extraction, who had a rented farm near Aberdeen. Like so many tenant farmers Mr Schense found it difficult to earn a livelihood, and the arrival of four more children added a severe burden. For the first eight years little help was forthcoming from the community, but in 1939 certain public-spirited people of Aberdeen decided to do something handsome for the quadruplets. They elected a "Schense Quadruplet Control Committee", whose object was to promote the general welfare and cultural development of the four children. A tag day during Education Week in 1939 brought in over $2,000 to finance the project. Had this help come sooner it would have been of greater benefit and would have made a great difference in the circumstances of the family. (Gardner and Newman 1944)

The Kaspar quadruplets were born May 9, 1936, in the Passaic General Hospital, Passaic, N.J. The parents are both German emigrés and the father a mechanic by trade. There are two older children, a boy of six and a half and a girl of eight years when the quadruplets were born. The family income was very small and the sudden addition of four more children threatened financial disaster. Help, however, was forthcoming from the mayor, who secured for the family several advertising contracts which have considerably improved their circumstances. It is thought that the worldwide publicity achieved by the Dionne quintuplets had much to do with increasing the interest of advertisers in this as in subsequent quadruplet births. The family income from advertising contracts has enabled the Kaspars not only to purchase the home they now occupy but has improved their situation in many other ways. (Gardner and Newman 1943a)

A story of that kind attaches to every higher multiple birth, relating to the provision of adequate space for the family, and to the massive demands for food and clothing over the years as parents have to buy four or more articles at a time in place of the usual outlay for one. This applies equally to furniture like cots and highchairs, and to the number of napkins or diapers that are needed. As one father of quins commented to the press, 'Remember, of course, we can't pass down clothes; everything has to be bought in fives' (*Woman's Own*, 5 January 1980).

Older children, relatives, friends and community agencies may offer help to the mother; it should be actively sought and readily accepted. However, it needs to be on a regular and continuing basis, and this can itself add strains to family life and friendships. When a one-child family becomes a six-child family following the birth of quins, the large group of same-age children presents much greater management problems than a family of six stepped in age and capable in part of caring for each other.

Even with adequate materiel the mother can become overwhelmed attempting to care for all her babies. Extra help to share in the household chores, especially initially, is usually necessary. (McFee *et al.* 1974)

Financial relief has come to some families from supply companies and appliance manufacturers and from gifts of food but this is often given in return for a degree of publicity that not all families are prepared to accept. In the case of the family mentioned above, the public expectation that multiple sets will receive such financial support had its unfortunate side.

The world thought that the arrival of the babies meant riches—newspapers vying with each other to buy exclusive rights to the quins' pictures, babyfood firms competing for the right to sponsor the children. But the money never came in. For months, the Inland Revenue couldn't believe that [the father] was telling the truth and he found himself having to write to publications asking them to confirm he hadn't signed lucrative contracts. (*Woman's Own*, 5 January 1980)

In most cases where such financial support has been reported, some outside agency, government department, community organization, service club or helpful citizen has sponsored an appeal or secured the services. Where the social and medical services can provide the mother with trained baby nurses for the period of her adjustment to the new demands this proves to be most helpful. An example of this was the help given to the family of the Good quads: two farmworker-type council houses were specially adapted for the family and two nurses from the preterm baby unit went home with them (Corner 1974). Two cases reported by

McFee *et al.* (1974) highlight these issues:

Caring for the needs of 4 infants under crowded circumstances was a big problem for this family. The husband's earnings, considering family size, approached the poverty line. Initially they resided in a small two-bedroom house where the quadruplets were housed in the dining room. During the year since the birth the family received many useful gifts although most were slow in arriving and the total did not completely meet their needs. A significant amount of money was also contributed which assisted in obtaining a larger house 1 year later. Although there were some voluntary homemaking services periodically, most of the housework and care of the infants was done by the patient with the help of her two older girls, ages 7 and 9. "Well child" care for the babies has been sporadic. At one point during their first year all the children were found to be anemic; otherwise, their health has been good. The patient more recently had a therapeutic abortion for a subsequent pregnancy which was believed to be a triplet gestation.

The problem of how to adequately care for 3 infants at one time—from the work-load and financial standpoints—hit this family very hard for a long time. They lived in a 3-bedroom house in a pleasant, recently developed Denver suburb. Income, although not in the poverty range, was low. Although the patient was discharged from the hospital soon after delivery it took several weeks for her to recover, primarily from mental depression due to the overwhelming thought of raising 3 children. The couple received essentially no help at any time either in the realm of baby supplies and equipment or of household help. This fact no doubt contributed to the mother's depression as she had been led to believe earlier that much help and gifts would be forthcoming. They were fortunate, however, in having a number of relatives living in the area who helped with household chores during the early weeks following the arrival of the babies at home. Firm determination by this couple of modest means to raise the infants with only their own resources has resulted in a successful outcome of these three girls, presently age 2 and developing normally.

The second of these cases is an important illustration because there are risks in higher multiple pregnancies which sometimes lead to a smaller group of babies surviving. If the needs of the family have to depend on the public wonder that accompanies an announcement of a large birth or the advertisers' interest which is dependent on that public wonder, then the loss of a baby can mean a lessening of that support. As the story suggests, the mother's adjustment to multiple birth had its own problems. In any case, public wonder is fickle, and today it is probably veering away from quadruplets toward sextuplet announcements.

The most successful support systems have been those which encouraged the family to cope and gave them help in doing so. In Gardner and Newman's (1944) account of the Schense quadruplets we see the problems created for family life by special provisions made for the multiple set:

The quadruplets were moved to Aberdeen, where they lived in comfortable quarters and were given everything necessary for their health and happiness, including exceptional educational opportunities. It was not long, however, before the Schense parents became dissatisfied with the arrangement. They feared, quite naturally, that a long separation from the rest of the family might bring about a breach between the quadruplets and their brothers and sisters on the farm, who were not invited to share the fine opportunities the quadruplets were enjoying. The result was that after spending a little more than a year as the guests of the Committee, the quadruplets returned to their home and have remained there ever since.

Another community effort was more successful:

. . we were informed that the The Galveston Chamber of Commerce had sponsored a successful drive to raise $20,000 for the purchase of a suitable home for the [Badgett] quads and their parents [and] that the family had moved into their new home in November, 1941. The quadruplets' third birthday was celebrated with a party on February 1, 1942, and all contributors to the house fund were invited as guests of honor. (Gardner and Newman 1942)

That help was still a little delayed. It is hard to get effective help to the families of multiple sets early, when they need it most.

In all the available reports, with the exception of the case quoted above, very little attention has been given to how the mothers of these children managed their child caring, feeding, sleeping, and general growth and development. In some countries paediatric supervision has been a continuing service; in others very little has been available especially for rural families. One mother breast-fed her babies, all four of them, for nine months. Whatever arrangements are made it becomes a full-time operation. Consider the hazards of taking four toddlers for a little picnic by a stream. As one wanders off toward some hazard how many hands are available to look after the other three while you chase the wanderer? The management problems alone force a kind of close-to-home pattern of interaction with the environment. If you don't have a car or can't drive and the preschool facilities are beyond the walking distance of your 3-year-olds, then without a community that rallies round to provide a transport roster you would not send your foursome to preschool. The child care problems for the parents of higher multiple sets are not insurmountable, as the reports of happy, healthy children in positively functioning families attest, but still they have a continuing presence.

In the face of such pressures it is realistic that parents who run the risk of multiple pregnancy should take out insurance against it and check their policies carefully to ensure adequate financial coverage.

The timing of the present pregnancy was planned and the patient had taken out an insurance policy against multiple pregnancy, after having had twins twice. (Fullerton *et al.* 1965)

(It is interesting to note that for many years insurance companies have had some of the best incidence figures on multiple births.)

However, most of the preparations for infant care, and the purchase of clothing and equipment will be delayed until after the birth of the babies when their survival is certain and when the family know how many new members they will be caring for. Neither the publicity, nor the purchasing can be fully prepared for ahead of time.

In recent years parent groups with professional help have been formed in some countries (see Appendix 2), often becoming registered charities. Some act as centres of information and give practical advice and help to families in need. A study of triplet and higher order births—aiming to find ways of improving the care and services provided for these children—is in progress in the United Kingdom under the auspices of the Office of Population Censuses and Surveys, the National Perinatal Epidemiology Unit and the Child Care and Development Group at the University of Cambridge.

The Goshen-Gottstein studies
Believing that 'there is no substitute for observations of family interactions within the natural habitat—the family—[where] the observer obtains rich qualitative

material that emerges spontaneously', Goshen-Gottstein (1976) investigated how mothers of twins, triplets and quadruplets divided their time between their different tasks at different stages of the infants' development. In a second study (Goshen-Gottstein 1980) she extended these observations to discover some of the basic issues facing the mother of multiple infants. The study included four families of quadruplets born in different parts of Israel. The families were visited monthly when the babies were 5 to 12 months old and then every two months to the age of 4 to 6 years.

There were many interesting findings. Particularly stressful times occurred when the children were ill, and at vacation time from school and nursery school. Bottle feeding was almost universal. Confining children to cribs, playpens or spaces was an energy saver. More so than singletons, multiple children became extremely competitive for their mother's attention, stayed close to her, and clamoured to be picked up or played with. This varied over time from child to child within the set.

Children were often treated as a unit in the service of efficiency which meant that there was an insensitivity to the individual scheduling of each child. This 'unitizing' of the set was also expressed in the language mothers tended to use. Quadruplets, who are harder to conceptualize as one than twins, tended to be divided into twos in arrangements for bedrooms, bathing, inside or outside play, and so on.

The mothers were attempting to cope with a situation for which they had not been readied. They needed to learn how to give themselves to four babies at once and care for each sensitively; how to occupy their children; how to be responsive to different children of the same age; and how to relate to each and all of them. Those who handled the situation best were those who previously had been nursery school or kindergarten teachers and who consequently were better prepared and trained to deal with more than one young child of the same age.

There were numerous dilemmas and task overloads which created stress. Goshen-Gottstein recommended that mothers of multiples should have opportunities to give vent to fears and negative feelings soon after the birth. She recommended supportive counselling both at the prenatal stage and after the birth, and training in how to individualize their interactions with the children (much as preschool teacher training does). In particular, mothers of identical sets need help before they can foster the growth of their infants as different people who need different experiences.

This is a rare example of a thorough observational study of higher multiple sets, conducted in the natural setting of the family, and which produced some useful guidelines for those in a position to act supportively to the parents of quads, quins and higher multiple sets.

Family relationships and group reactions
Obviously the family relationships of a higher multiple set would make a potentially instructive subject for study, especially if they were observed over a period of time. A child psychologist involved in well-baby checks and developmental guidance would be in an advantageous position to gain family consent for such a study. (Having said this, it must be stressed that any such approach, and subsequent

investigation, should only be made with strict regard to ethical standards and to the individual rights of the children and their parents or guardians.)

How do the members of a multiple set behave toward each other? Patterns of interactions would vary with a number of factors including zygosity, family circumstances and family styles of interactions. Collation of brief references from various reports suggests that any hypothesis on the effects of being members of a same-age sibling set of three or more should be related to a particular set or should be very carefully checked on several.

The Morlok girls had no brothers or sisters, meaning a less complex situation than occurs in larger families. Gardner and Newman (1943*b*) noted that 'group-of-four' behaviour when the girls acted as a unit was less evident than in the other quadruplet sets they studied. The girls showed more of a tendency toward normal individual behaviour. There were no siblings to unite against in defence of group rights.

The separation of the Dionne quins from their siblings for many years perhaps allowed scope for individual differences to emerge. As Blatz (1939) reported:

[At 3 years] the children have shown . . . decided and individual traits of social behaviour. It will be interesting to watch how they respond to the new social contacts which they will inevitably make as their social behaviour expands to include other children.

The MZ Auckland quads (see Chapter 5, p. 73) by comparison were more like the set of twins studied by Gesell and Thompson (1941) who 'equalized the influence of their own mutual companionship' and maintained similar personality characteristics. As a group they were mutually supportive. According to their responses to the Bene–Anthony Family Relations Test* (*personal data*), they lived in a home of unusually positive interactions. Most exchanges between family members were low-keyed but positive, and most of the negatively toned responses were placed in a 'throw-away' category not allocated to any family member. Some covert competition between two of the quads was expressed in this projective test situation. Two other personal and social adjustment measures (see p. 74) indicated the same quiet, positive, somewhat passive mode of interaction with their social environment for each of the sisters, but with an indication that two pairs within the group were reacting with some individual differences. At 12 years of age re-administration of the Bene–Anthony test in modified group form (Clay and Oates 1984) showed that the same positive family tone of interaction prevailed. By comparing each quad with national survey results for this age-group, four separate checks on this conclusion were made. The quads reported more positive interactions with family members than other children of the same age (higher positive ratings to parents, outgoing positive feelings to brothers and sisters, and negative statements mostly seen as applying to 'nobody'). Their two elder brothers did not collect negative allocations typically given to siblings but the sisters gave each other as many negative and positive statements as other children of their age

---

*The Bene–Anthony Family Relations Test (Children's Version) quantifies subjects' feelings toward relatives, and assesses the attitudes they perceive relatives show toward them, by means of a set of alternative emotions or attitudes printed onto cards. (*Catalogue of Tests for Educational and Clinical Psychologists.* Windsor: NFER, p. 33.)

give to siblings. There were signs of individual differences among the sisters: one expressed a strong attachment to one older brother; another had polarized her relationships with her parents, giving positive responses to the mother and negative responses to the father. Overall, a division of family relationships and roles was suggested that would not be unusual in any six-sibling family.

Whether a group functions as a unit, in pairs or as individuals depends on the family environment, the social setting and in particular past social learning. By 5 years of age the Lawson quintuplets (also born in New Zealand) had learned certain social behaviours because they were five same-age children growing up together. The following comments are from my notes:

Each was skilled in subtle ways of drawing attention to him or herself, a survival strategy in an outgoing multiple group. When I paid a visit to their school for regular observations and I asked one who had finished working with me to tell one of the other siblings to come to me, I was met with a polite but very, very firm retort, "I'll send you Billy." Billy was a chosen friend deliberately selected to exclude the other siblings.

They were well schooled in controlling children of their own age. When they were still novices in the New Entrant classroom at 5 years the teacher found she could ask any one of them to stand in front of her class of 15 to 20 new entrants seated on the mat, get them in order and start some kind of group activity. They were practised in managing children of their own age.

This set were outgoing initiators of their own experiences, different in appearance, different in personality, strongly individual in social interactions and attention seeking.

Some reports emphasize stable pairings within multiple sets, as with the Morlok quads:

The two larger girls play more often together, while the two smaller tend to keep together in play and in friendships. This pairing may have been initiated by and accentuated by the fact that from an early age the two pairs mentioned have had two separate bedrooms. So there may be nothing very difficult for the psychologist to explain in this group-within-the-group behavior. (Gardner and Newman 1943*b*)

Other sets form groupings of convenience, like the 5-year-old quins who had developed very effective strategies for defeating parents' control measures by forming active 'gangs' of three, four or five as the occasion warranted. The power of the group has also been used in school settings (Clay, *unpublished case studies*).

Multiple sets are often split into separate classes on entry to school, either for sake of convenience or in order to encourage individuality (see, for instance, Fig. 2.2, p. 20). Whereas some sets will respond well to this, in others it will be resisted, as with the set of quads interviewed by *You* magazine (8 July 1984):

'They split us up at school,' remembers Marie bitterly, 'because they said they could not tell us apart. They made us wear a big initial letter on our uniforms—and then still got it wrong.' 'We minded this isolation,' adds Patsy. 'We thought there must be something wrong with us to be so marked out.' Being thus separated is one of the factors of being a quad that the girls resented most. As if in defiance, they would regroup in the playground and play intently with each other.

The overriding public reaction (often strongly reinforced in the family) is to the group set-up as, for instance, with the Good quads:

Until they left school, the family, the local community and the general public treated the children as a group and invariably included the older sister in all their private and public activities, but their parents had considerable insight into their individual aptitudes and interests. They were dressed alike, and were always given similar treats and toys. (Corner 1974)

This public response to the unusual multiple nature of the group is reinforced by publicity and in certain cases by training for public performances, as in this report of the Morlok quads:

They sing together as a quartette and are said by good judges to be excellent in their harmony. They are also being trained to dance as a team and in this they show considerable promise. (Gardner and Newman 1943*b*)

How early do the members of a multiple set recognize their group characteristics? My observations of an MZ set of triplets at 3 years suggested that, although each child could clearly identify the others by correct name (a task on which I failed miserably), their attempts to relate to me were markedly individual, and each used me to transmit a message to a sister alongside them. There was no three-way conversation. In some families it may take a little longer for multiples to learn to work as individuals in a group than for different aged siblings.

A Milwaukee mother of a three-girl set, aged five, commented amusingly, "When they go outdoors and can't find their friends, the three run back and say, 'We haven't got anyone to play with.'" (Scheinfeld 1968)

Psychologists interested in small-group dynamics would find the detailed study of higher multiple sets fascinating. Specific questions of sex role learning could be of particular interest, for if one is the only boy or the only girl in a group of same-age siblings the press of learning opportunities may well be predominantly from the opposite sex (though of course this will depend to a great extent on family circumstances and any special or different treatment given to that individual). One caution for the researcher in this area is that there are so many different possibilities for inter-relationships that linear-type hypotheses or prior conceptions are likely to be unproductive. At least initially, study will need to be based on detailed observation and recording of what occurs.

Do children of the same age living in the same social environment manifest the same traits? Personal/social development is not only a response to the physical surroundings and the people in it but also a function of the individual's own response to the environment. This response colours every subsequent reaction and thus grows on itself (Blatz 1939). Case reports suggest increasing individual differences in personal/social development as the children move toward adolescence. That would seem appropriate.

Adult life

The Keys quads were the first set to be studied in adult life as they reached their college years in the period of high interest in plural births in the 1930s. They had the double distinction of being the first surviving set in the USA to receive wide publicity and the first recorded set to graduate from university (Gardner and Newman 1940*b*).

The developmental outcomes of the Good quads were summarized by Corner (1974) as follows.

The family travelled widely in Britain and abroad on sponsored holidays and the girls also showed enterprise with independent travel. On leaving school they established their individuality as shown by different hair styles, clothes and leisure activities, and their childhood rôle as quadruplets was resented. Although there were strong emotional ties with their fairly large extended family in the neighbourhood, the girls trained for careers away from home.

Bridget became secretary to a lawyer, married at 20 years a training college lecturer and lives in a country town near the farm.

Frances trained as a groom for horses and married a local farmer during her twentieth year. Two pregnancies resulted in normal sons, birth weights 6 lb 12 oz, and 5 lb 12 oz.

Elizabeth went as a nursery nurse to California, U.S.A., and Boston, Mass., and also attended technical college part-time for further studies. After returning home in 1969 for the 21st birthday celebration she continued as a nursery nurse with a British family in West Germany and became engaged to be married to a soldier in Autumn 1972.

Jennifer trained in kennel management and is employed in a large dog breeding establishment.

The mother of the quadruplets was intelligent, active and had many interests outside the home. Unfortunately she was unable to control excessive obesity and heavy smoking and in October 1971 she died from a sudden subarachnoid hemorrhage. The father is still alive and healthy. The elder sister is married and has two healthy children.

The life-span developmental psychology of higher multiples is rarely recorded. The sad exception is the life of the Dionnes, still dominating the book and media markets with the riches-to-poverty life stories of five children who grew up in difficult circumstances. Berton's book (*The Dionne Years: A Thirties Melodrama*) and a TV documentary shown recently in New Zealand report circumstances no worse than those encountered by many adults. It is a media message that hangs like a cloud over higher multiples seeking a normal life. The message is pessimistic: problems and defeat in the search for happiness. In this sense the public preoccupation with the first living set of five has done little to help and much to endanger the happiness of other multiples. Again, the adult story of the Genain quads as reported by Rosenthal (1963) is an important psychiatric study of mental illness, yet it contributes nothing to our understanding of how to normalize development.

There are isolated developmental reports of quads with positive life outcomes, in particular the long article by Schlaginhaufen (1940) on the Gehri quads, born in 1880 and still alive at 60 years, and one by Nowalowski (1974) on the MZ Wroclaw quads, the only reported all-male set, whose development was followed to 18 years. I was fortunate in 1982 to correspond with the 47-year-old Johnson quads (see Catalogue, 6 March 1935) and their 81-year-old mother, and more recently with the Alexanders and their 22-year-old quadruplet daughters (see Catalogue, 2 September 1967). Such contacts yield anecdotal data which is interesting but does not add up to a cohesive view of the developmental psychology of higher multiple sets in adult life.

5
STUDYING MULTIPLE SETS: OLD AND NEW DEVELOPMENTAL REPORTS

Developmental studies of higher multiples have rarely been extensive or innovative. The scant evidence on psychological variables in quadruplets is reported in this chapter, supplemented with some data from twins and from the Dionne quintuplets. Where studies have repeatedly used the same analysis with several sets of multiples, only examples or comparative data are reported. The only quadruplet sets for whom there are reports covering substantial sections of their lives are the Keys quads, the Good quads and the Genain quads (three all-girl sets) and the Wroclaw quads (all males). The MZ Auckland quads, mentioned in Chapter 4 (pp. 42–43), were studied by the present author from the age of 3 years to 7 years 3 months, and original data from test and behaviour records for this set also are reported in this chapter.

Physical growth
Birthweight in multiple pregnancies
From historical records, most quadruplets weighed between 1250 and 1800g at birth; around one-third weighed between 900 and 1250g, and very few weighed more than 2250g.

McKeown and Record (1952) suggested that the maternal organism is capable of supporting fetal growth in plural pregnancy without prejudice to the individual fetus until the total weight of babies and birth membranes reaches about 7 lbs. (3100g). They believed that later growth retardation was determined by the inability of the prenatal environment fully to meet the fetal needs rather than an inability of the fetuses to maintain their growth rate. They examined fetal growth in 22,454 singleton, 325 twin, 249 triplet and 27 quadruplet maternities. The rate of growth slowed for quadruplets from about 26 weeks; for triplets from 27 weeks; for twins from 30 weeks; and for singletons from 36 weeks. Ounsted and Ounsted (1973) summarized the situation: individual fetuses in multiple litters are slow-grown; the larger the litter, the earlier the deceleration begins.

Mean birthweights for singletons, twins, triplets and quadruplets in the McKeown and Record survey were, respectively, 7.43, 5.27, 4.00 and 3.07 lbs. (3370, 2390, 1814 and 1393g). Mean litter weights were 7.43, 10.53, 12.00 and 12.28 lbs. (3370, 4776, 5443 and 5570g). The mean gestation times were, respectively, 280.5, 261.6, 246.8 and 236.8 days. The early onset of labour in higher order pregnancies may be due to the amount of distension that the uterus will tolerate during the last weeks of gestation.

More recently, with improved prenatal care and nutrition, higher birthweights are becoming more common. In addition, advances in natal and neonatal care have meant that many more very low-birthweight babies are surviving.

TABLE 5.I
Correlations of heights and weights in MZ and DZ twins in two studies

Study	MZ		DZ	
	Height	Weight	Height	Weight
Husén (1959)	0.89	0.81	0.59	0.56
Shields (1962)	0.94	0.80	0.44	0.56

Influence of sex and zygosity on birthweight
Zygosity and sex have been related to birthweight in twins. In a series of 528 unselected newborn twin pairs of known zygosity, Corney *et al.* (1972) found that:
* on average, MZ twins weighed less than DZ twins when sex and placentation were taken into account;
* the difference remained when MZ and DZ twins were equated for body length and gestation time;
* MZ male twins weighed more than MZ female twins.

The authors analysed the sets according to whether they were monochorionic (MC) or dichorionic (DC). MZ twins weighed about the same whether MC or DC, and in either case they tended to be lighter than DZ twins. The authors were also able to demonstrate that all three types of twins (MZ-MC, MZ-DC, DZ-DC) had similar gestation times.

Growth trends
Do children of plural births, who begin life lighter, compensate for their low birthweight in later childhood or does growth retardation persist? Twins in Drillen's Scottish survey (1964) remained below national norms for both height and weight at the age of 5 years, and a large sample of 873 Swedish male twins studied by Husén (1959) at 18 years had a mean height which was 1.3cm below that of singleton conscripts for military service. However, more recent studies (Wilson 1974, 1979; Ljung *et al.* 1977) have shown a greater catch-up growth in twins than previously recorded. In two British studies MZ twins were found to be shorter than DZ twins (Shields 1962, Corney *et al.* 1972). In Husén's sample the MZ twins were on average 1kg lighter than the DZ twins; in Shields' sample there was a greater difference.

If body build were genetically determined one would expect greater concordance within MZ twin sets as compared to DZ twins. Two studies (Husén 1959, Shields 1962) have confirmed this, finding higher correlations in MZ twins for both height and weight (Table 5.I). The differences among Husén's samples at adolescence were small, whereas Shields' samples showed greater differences, probably due to the greater age distribution.

Studies of physical growth in quadruplets
THE KEYS QUADRUPLETS
An early and extensive study of the physical growth of the Keys quads was made by Spier (1928). The set consisted of an MZ pair (Roberta and Mona) and a DZ pair

TABLE 5.II
Physical measurements of the Keys quadruplets at 12 years*

	MZ		DZ	
	Roberta	Mona	Mary	Leota
Order of birth	1st	2nd	3rd	4th
Weight at birth (kg)	1.6	2.0	1.8	1.4
Height				
Standing (cm)	151.4	155.9	151.4	145.7
Sitting (cm)	75.3	77.4	75.5	74.9
Length				
Span of arms (cm)	149.2	150.5	148.6	143.0
Shoulder to elbow (cm)	L 29.0	L 31.3	L 30.2	L 27.8
	R 28.8	R 30.7	R 31.8	R 27.3
Elbow to finger tip (cm)	L 40.3	L 40.9	L 40.2	L 38.0
	R 40.4	R 41.5	R 40.3	R 38.8
Leg to top of hips (cm)	L 95.6	L 97.0	L 93.0	L 89.4
	R 95.9	R 96.3	R 93.2	R 89.4
Face (cm)	10.6	11.0	11.1	10.7
Width				
Shoulder (cm)	31.5	32.2	32.3	31.0
Hips (cm)	24.1	24.9	26.2	23.2
Face (cm)	11.4	11.1	11.2	11.3
Wrist (cm)	L 4.6	L 4.9	L 4.7	L 4.6
	R 4.7	R 4.8	R 4.9	R 4.6
Chest width (cm)	22.3	22.3	25.2	22.2
Chest depth (cm)	16.7	17.9	16.4	15.6
Head diameter				
Anteroposterior (cm)	18.3	18.2	18.7	17.8
Transverse (cm)	13.8	14.0	14.1	13.6
Height (cm)	12.3	13.0	11.8	11.6
Circumference				
Head and hair (cm)	52.6	52.6	53.0	51.1
Chest (cm)	68.8	71.8	69.0	63.5
Hips (cm)	71.0	73.5	76.0	66.2
Wrist (cm)	L 13.0	L 13.3	L 14.2	L 13.1
	R 13.5	R 13.5	R 14.1	R 13.0
Upper arm (cm)	L 19.0	L 19.8	L 19.7	L 18.4
	R 19.0	R 19.8	R 19.6	R 18.2
Upper arm, flexed (cm)	L 20.3	L 20.6	L 20.8	L 19.1
	R 20.2	R 20.7	R 20.4	R 18.9
Weight (with light indoor clothing and without shoes) (kg)	36.7	40.4	43.9	33.1
Indices				
Sitting–standing	49.7	49.7	49.6	51.2
Cephalic	75.5	76.9	75.3	76.5
Chest	74.8	80.1	65.0	70.3
Growth of hair: axillae	None	None	None	None

Erupted teeth
  Roberta   Full permanent dentition except third molars
  Mona   Full permanent dentition, including upper left third molar only
  Mary   As Roberta
  Leota   Permanent dentition alone, except third molars and upper left first biscuid, the canines being erupted, but below the occlusal plane

*Adapted from Spier (1928).

(Mary and Leota). To enable the reader to make MZ–DZ comparisons, measurements taken when the girls were 12 years old are given in Table 5.II.

GARDNER AND NEWMAN REPORTS

In a series of studies of quadruplets, these authors used a short list of physical measures and characteristics for within-set comparisons. The three examples given in Table 5.III describe different types of quadruplets—a DZ set of singleton plus 'triplets', an MZ set and a QZ set.

THE GOOD QUADRUPLETS

Similarities and differences in the physical measurements of the Good quads (a TZ set made up of MZ and DZ twin pairs) were reported by their paediatrician in a longitudinal study (Corner 1974). They provide some interesting comparisons (Table 5.IV). Note the shift in the height measurements of the MZ pair between birth and 1 year.

THE WROCLAW QUADRUPLETS

The MZ Polish quads of Wroclaw are the only all-male MZ set reported in the literature. They were studied by scientists in several research institutions at different stages in their lives. One of the four boys suffered one-sided paresis and deafness, probably due to injury during labour; as a result he lived apart from the rest of the family during some of his growing years. He was taught to speak and overcame the birth injuries to a great extent. Nowakowski (1974) compared the development of these quads up to the age of 3 years with the development of four (randomly selected) boys from the same State Home for Babies in which they lived. The measures used were not explained in that report, but assuming that some composite measure of body build was used to take both height and weight into account, certain important features emerge.
★ The quads were very small when first studied.
★ They all moved toward normal levels with somewhat similar acceleration and against the normative trend which dips gradually.
★ They were not very different at 3 years, although they developed to that age on different growth schedules.
★ Even the injured boy, K, showed a pattern which 'stubbornly' strove at compensation for the arrest (Nowakowski 1974).

By comparison, the control children (two of normal birthweight and two of low birthweight) were arrested in physical development with two falling behind and two gaining by 3 years, but all below normal development.

Nowakowski reported that the development of the three non-injured quads during their school years would be represented on a graph *by a single line*, because the plotted points were so close together. Their body build was very similar, slim and lean. They were somewhat below average in growth but the deficit was negligible by 18 years of age. Only 10 measurements were available for the fourth boy and a fair comparison could not be made with the other three. Although smaller and lighter for most of his childhood, by the end of adolescence he had attained an identical weight and was only 4cm shorter than his brothers.

TABLE 5.III
Physical characteristics of three sets of quadruplets

BADGETT, 1:0 yrs. (Gardner and Newman 1942)	MZ 'triplets'			Singleton
	Jeraldine	Joyce	Jeannette	Joan
Standing height (cm)	70	69.5	74	74
Sitting height (cm)	44	43	43.5	45.7
Weight (kg)	8.6	8.6	8.6	9.8
Head length (cm)	14.7	14.6	14.7	15.3
Head width (cm)	11.2	10.6	10.7	10.6
Cephalic index	76.1	72.6	72.7	69.4
Hair colour	Very fair	Very fair	Very fair	Light brown
Hair character	Fine and curly	Fine and curly	Fine and curly	Fine but straight
Eye colour	Light blue flecked with brown	Same as Jeraldine	Same as Jeraldine	Grayish blue, no brown flecks
No. of teeth	5	4	4	4

MORLOK, 10:3 yrs. (Gardner and Newman 1943b)	MZ			
	Edna	Wilma	Sarah	Helen
Standing height (cm)	133	129	132	126
Sitting height (cm)	67	66	66	65
Weight (kg)	24.5	23.1	24.0	22.5
Head length (cm)	17.7	16.5	17.7	17
Head width (cm)	12.5	12.2	12.2	12
Cephalic index	70.7	73.9	70.6	70.6
Eye colour	light brown, some flecking	same	same	same
Hair	light candy	same	same	same
Hair texture	fine, straight	same	same	same
Skin colour	fair	same	same	same
Teeth	even, no cavities	same	same	same

SCHENSE, 13:0 yrs. (Gardner and Newman 1944)	QZ			
	Joan	Jean	James	Jay
Standing height (cm)	132	134	137	140
Sitting height (cm)	69	71	72	73
Head length (cm)	16.7	17.5	16.5	17.7
Head width (cm)	13.0	14.0	13.2	14.5
Cephalic index	78.8	80.0	80.0	81.9
Eye colour	hazel	light blue	hazel	light brown
Hair colour	light brown	light blond	medium brown	light brown
Skin colour	slightly dark	very fair	sun tan	slightly dark
Dentition	very irregular, 13 out	regular, smaller than others	irregular, larger than others	regular but widely spaced
Handedness	right	right	right	left
Hair whorl	clockwise	same	same	same

TABLE 5.IV
Physical growth records for the Good quadruplets*

Age		MZ		DZ	
		Francis	Elizabeth	Bridget	Jennifer
Birth	Weight (kg)	1.82	2.00	1.75	1.78
	Height (cm)	40.5	44.5	40.5	39.0
1 yr.	Weight (kg)	11.0	11.2	8.9	8.4
	Height (cm)	74	75	70	70
21 yrs.	Weight (kg)	54.0	53.0	55.0	53.5
	Height (cm)	170.7	170.2	166.0	177.8

*Adapted from Corner (1974).

Nowakowski concluded:

The impression is acquired that not only body height, but also body weight and other physical and mental traits, are to a much greater extent under genetic control than it is generally assumed, and that genetic factors prevail in the shaping of the phenotype.

THE DIONNE QUINTUPLETS

Physical growth data for the Dionnes were reported longitudinally and with normative comparison (Dafoe 1934, 1936, 1937, 1940; Blatz 1937, 1939; Blatz et al. 1937; MacArthur and Dafoe 1939). Plotted against normal female child growth they showed continuing gain on a slope which was at first accelerated but which settled to the normal rate of increase around the age of 1 year. Height and weight shifted within the normal range up to 5 years. At almost all times they maintained their birthweight order. They rose above mean weight levels after 3 years and made rapid gains in height between 4 and 5 years. MacArthur and Dafoe plotted the average differences between all 10 possible pairings of the quins for both height and weight up to 5 years. The differences were greatest at 8 to 9 days and were at their lowest level after 2 years, with weight more variable than height.

Ossification of bones

Pryor (1936, 1939, 1948) explored the hypothesis that variation in the sequence of ossification of bones is a heritable trait. He was interested in the sequence in which the eight carpal bones of the hand begin ossification. This may occur at different times, so there is opportunity for a vast number of patterns. Sometimes an extra epiphysis is found at the central end of the second metacarpal bone. Pryor found this extra bone present in the hands of both members of a set of MZ twins, and in all the members of two sets of MZ triplets and one set of MZ quadruplets. Pryor's data for three quadruplet sets of different zygosity revealed the following contrasts.

★ The Perricone quadruplets showed varying patterns which could not have come from the chromosomes of a single zygote. They were genotypically different, supporting the hypothesis of a QZ origin (see also Gardner and Newman 1940*a*).

★ The Schense quadruplets, judged on somewhat incomplete data for carpal

ossification, could have been trizygotic—the boys could be MZ twins, the girls were not. The evidence from the boys was not convincing of MZ origin but presented nothing contrary to it.
★ For the Morlok quadruplets—MZ by any other criteria—any hand could represent the entire eight (except for a slight variation in one girl's hands). All four had an extra epiphysis on the central end of the second metacarpal bone. This is a very rare occurrence and a striking demonstration of the similarity of the eight hands.

Pryor was searching for a means of confirming the zygosity of multiple sets. Because of the proven usefulness of blood analyses, which were begun about the same period, bone ossification is today of little interest.

Dentition
Reports on higher multiple sets referring to similarities and differences in dentition timing and sequence have tended to be isolated descriptions which do not show clearly the amount of variation (*e.g.* Brintle 1931, Kaminska 1974). Dentition status in the Keys quads at 12 years was reported by Spier (1928) (see Table 5.II).

Physical resemblance
Brief mention must be made of the physical likenesses within MZ pairs or sets. With the progress of science, blood analysis techniques became highly reliable indicators of zygosity and other tests were discarded. Psychological variables shrank to one question, used in a study by Cederlöf *et al.* (1961). They asked adult twins, 'When you were growing up were you as alike as two peas in a pod or was there only a family likeness?' Where both members of a twin pair answered the question consistently, there was a 95 per cent agreement with zygosity data.

Cohen *et al.* (1973, 1975) asked parents of 94 MZ and 61 DZ twins 10 questions about similarities on physical characteristics, and about identity and confusion. MZ and DZ twins were clearly separated on the basis of the total set of answers. Information was in error in fewer than 3 per cent of cases and approximated quite well the results of blood typing for zygosity assignment.

Such approaches can only be used as a probe or check, and cannot be used to confirm zygosity.

Health histories
Health histories have occasionally been reported. Brintle (1931) provided brief histories of the Keys quads to the age of 11 years, while more detailed histories were provided for the Good quads by Corner (1974)—notes on their growth to age 21 years have been shown in Table 5.IV.

Gross and fine motor development
Despite medical interest in multiple sets there have been few studies of their motor development. From twin studies Anastasi (1979) concluded that there is a substantial genetic component in sensory, perceptual and motor behaviour. Training studies by Hilgard (1933) of a set of MZ twins at 4½ years demonstrated

that genetic control is greater over simple motor tasks and less over more complex tasks. The twins were found to be highly similar on preliminary tests of intelligence, vocabulary, drawing, memory, handedness, footedness and motor speed. They displayed differences on perseveration tests. When the experiment began the twins were well-matched on motor tests of cutting, ring-tossing, and on walking-boards of 2, 4 and 6cm width. Special practice produced considerable rises in performance scores and what appeared like an initial gain for the twin whose practice began later settled back to similar performance of both twins at follow-up tests three to six months later.

There were follow-up differences according to the particular task given. Performance on the walking boards showed no loss but continued to show a slight gain. Loss at the end of the follow-up period was shown in ring-tossing activity. Cutting did not show comparable patterns of progress because 'an individual technique produced a consistent difference so that the delayed twin never equalled the score of her earlier-practised sister'. (Hilgard 1933)

It seems that handwriting is also too complex a task to be subject to genetic control in any direct sense. In studies by Galton (1875) and Husén (1959) the differences in handwriting between MZ twins were as great as those between DZ twins.

Tests of psychomotor development were given to the 'Danzig quins'* once a month from 3 months of age. Their physical progress is illustrated pictorially in Figure 5.1, and the 'developmental quotient' scores are recorded in Table 5.V.

At the age of 3 months a retardation of psychomotor development was found in all children, although it was not too far advanced, except in Piotr. This retardation varied within the limits of 2-3 weeks, and that of Piotr amounted to more than 1 month.

At the age of 4 months two children, Adam and Ewa, had results within the limits of normality. Adam had better results; this is probably in connection with his better physical condition. Two infants, Roman and Agnieszka, showed a slight retardation by some 2 weeks in comparison with chronological age, and the values of development quotients (DQ) approached the limits of normality. Piotr continued to be backward in his psychomotor development by 1 month approximately.

At the age of 5 months all infants obtained results within the limits of normality. Adam and Ewa were in the upper limit, and Piotr in the lower one.

At the age of 7 months Adam and Ewa's psychomotor DQ values corresponded to the upper limit of mean values. The rapid progress of Piotr's physical development in that month found its parallel in a considerable acceleration of the rate of psychomotor development. For the first time Piotr's DQ exceeded 100 (good norm).

When the infants concluded their 12th month, i.e., at the age of 1 year, the developmental age of all children exceeded the chronological age. This means that DQs achieved values over 100. The differences in the rate of psychomotor development between the children increased. Adam and Ewa considerably outpaced their siblings achieving DQs at a level above the average (113). (Bogdanowicz 1974)

---

*The 'Danzig quins' (family name: Rychert) were born in Gdansk, Poland, on 15 May 1971 (Danzig at that time being the more commonly known English equivalent name for Gdansk). The mother, who was 32 years old, already had two sons of 6 and 7 years, and a further pregnancy, in 1964, had ended in abortion. She had had no hormonal treatment. The quins were born at 33 weeks gestation by assisted vaginal delivery, with birthweights ranging from 1280 to 2000g (Metler and Rudzinski 1974). Placental analysis (Metler *et al.* 1974) and blood groupings (Raszeja and Krueger 1974) suggested that they were of quintovular origin.

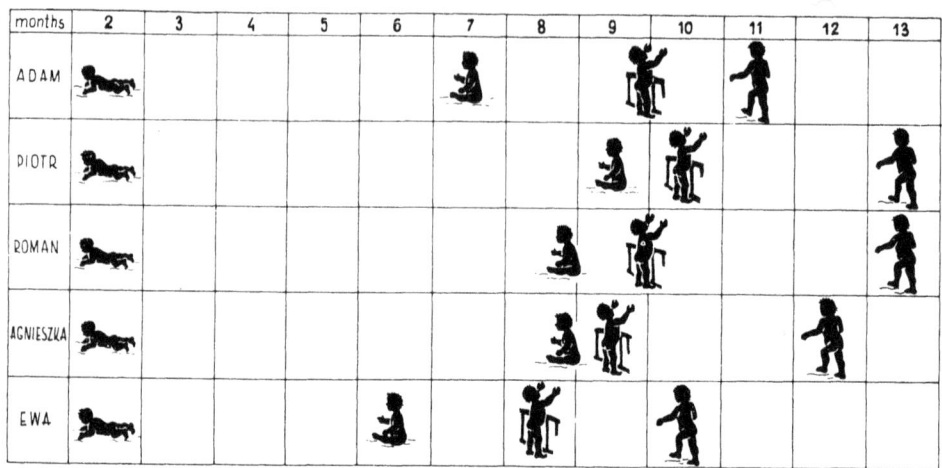

Fig. 5.1. Physical development of the Danzig quintuplets in the first year of life (Kaminska 1974).

TABLE 5.V

Psychological follow-up of the Danzig quintuplets in their first year of life*

Age (months)	DQ values (Brunet–Lézine scale of Psychomotor Development)				
	Adam	Piotr	Roman	Agnieszka	Ewa
4	97	72	87	85	90
5	110	94	·100	100	106
6	110	96	101	100	105
7	110	100	101	101	108
8	110	100	102	107	110
9	110	100	102	107	110
10	109	100	100	103	110
11	110	100	100	103	110
12	113	103	100	103	113

*Bogdanowicz (1974).

In that report it is possible to see some of the advantages of a study of a multizygotic set growing up in the same environment and under the same rearing schedules.

★ The rate of psychomotor development was different for each of the infants.
★ The different developmental sequences all served to bring the early retardation up to normal or average levels.
★ The pace of development varied in different aspects of motor development. (Adam developed the fastest in motor development of the hands and in sight–movement co-ordination, while Ewa was ahead in body posture and locomotion.)

TABLE 5.VI
Proportions of left-handed twins, and of twins discordant for handedness*, in four study groups

Study	Left-handed		Discordant	
	MZ %	DZ %	MZ %	DZ %
Husén (1959)	6	6	12	12
Zazzo (1960)	16.1	12.9	24.4	22.1
Shields (1962)	10	12	17	18
Koch (1966)	15	14	—	—

*One twin right-handed, the other left-handed.

In spite of individual differences the psychomotor development of the quins proceeded at a normal rate and rhythm after making up for the initial deficiencies resulting from preterm birth, low birthweight, multiple pregnancy, and the incubator and special care conditions of the perinatal period (see Dziedziuszko and Krywko 1974).

Handedness and lateral inversions
Most researchers (with the exception of Husén) agree in reporting a higher incidence of left-handedness among both MZ and DZ twins than among singletons, but the percentages differ substantially from study to study (Table 5.VI). All agree that there is no difference in incidence between MZ and DZ twins. This disposes of many hypotheses, without suggesting any new ones. The higher incidence of left-handedness cannot, for instance, be explained for MZ twins by the way in which the cells split. The hypotheses favoured are environmental ones. Prenatal environment (crowding and position) may have some influence, and learning in the postnatal environment may favour one hand more often than in singleton children. There is little indication of what one may expect among higher multiple sets.

'Lateral inversion' refers to the asymmetry that occurs in individuals in handedness, hair whorls, dentition and dermatoglyphics (see Price 1950). Some twins show mirror-imaging for some or all of these characteristics. The term is also used for major asymmetries such as placement of the body organs. Asymmetries occur less often in dichorionic than in monochorionic twins and most often in conjoined twins. The phenomenon has been attributed to disturbances of the twinning process, or to the timing of cell division, occurring in cases where division occurs later rather than earlier. Price concluded that lateral inversions would be of limited diagnostic value in studies of handedness, handwriting and analagous variables, and in cases of doubtful zygosity when blood tests cannot be used.

To determine the handedness of the MZ Auckland quads at entry to school, they were observed in rotation for 10-second intervals during one hour of self-selected play activities in the classroom. One girl used or led with the left hand without exception, two consistently used the right hand, while the other used or led with either hand (*personal data*). Their subsequent hand use in approaching written texts in reading is reported later (see pp. 62–63).

Lenneberg (1966) advanced the hypothesis that language acquisition, maturation and handedness are intimately related; however, Mittler (1971) compared right- and left-handed twins on the Illinois Test of Psycholinguistic Abilities and found no significant differences.

General intelligence

In large-scale studies, the intelligence test scores of twins have been lower than those of singletons (Scottish Council for Educational Research 1953, Zazzo 1960, Record *et al.* 1970, Wilson and Harping 1972). The differences are not due to age, family structure or environment, or to the subgroup of twins with unusually low scores.

Because early studies emphasized genetic factors it is important to note some recent criticisms and debate. Lewontin (1975) claimed that simple comparisons of MZ and DZ twins assume that the amount of shared environmental experience is, on average, the same regardless of zygosity. Two studies relate to this issue. Foch and Plomin (1980) suggested that environmental factors may have considerable influence on test scores because they operate within families to make family members different from one another more than they make them similar to one another; while Fischbein (1977) argued that the contribution of genetic variance to intelligence test scores may be larger in a more stimulating environment and proportionately smaller in a disadvantaged environment.

In studies of MZ quadruplets environmental factors are of particular interest because hypotheses concerning their influence can be tested effectively using children of the same age and genetics, growing up in what appears to be the same environment and with the same range of experiences.

In a recent study of low-birthweight, preterm higher multiples (Krall *et al.* 1980), quadruplets and quintuplets were tested at regular three-monthly intervals during the first two years of life, using the Bayley Mental and Motor Scales, and their performance was contrasted with that of low-birthweight, preterm singletons. Mental and Motor Development indices were significantly correlated with birthweight, whether or not scores were adjusted for gestational age ($r=0.59$ to 0.83, $p<0.05$ to 0.01). After such adjustment, scores were in the average range at every interval. Unadjusted scores showed positive acceleration with age, and both quads and quins appeared to catch up to the average by about 2 years.

Intelligence among higher multiples: case reports

The validity of intelligence test scores has been studied extensively in recent years and it is not inappropriate now to view them as good indicators of general achievement (Vernon 1960).

The Keys quads developed normally but differently (Brintle 1931). At 12 years Roberta, Mona and Leota had scores which were considerably above average for children of that age, and which were strikingly similar. Mary's scores were almost exactly at the average and there was a consistent difference between her scores and the scores of the other three. (The Keys quads were a TZ set, Roberta and Mona being MZ 'twins'.)

The MZ Genain quads showed consistent but small differences on mental ability tests (Bayley 1963). At 10 years 3 months they were doing well in school having nearly completed Grade 4. Teachers reported that their work was careful and painstaking and none of them stood out from the others in achievement or ability. Some minor differences were recorded on the Stanford–Binet (Form L), the Army Beta Performance Test and the Stanford Achievement Tests. In comparison, the Schense quads, a QZ set, showed greater differences at 9 years 7 months on the Stanford–Binet and Army Beta tests (Table 5.VII).

Longitudinal testing
Some studies of higher multiple sets have traced cognitive growth over a period of time. Longitudinal data will be reported from one set of MZ quads and from the (MZ) Dionne quins.

The Dionnes were given developmental tests on 13 occasions between the ages of 17 and 35 months (Blatz and Millichamp 1937, Blatz 1939). Scores for all five children increased over that period. The overall levels of scoring were similar, but individual differences were found (Fig. 5.2) and a rank for ability remained almost undisturbed (Fig. 5.3).

In contrast to these consistent rankings, longitudinal data for the MZ Auckland quads, for six administrations of intelligence tests between the ages of 3 years 1 month and 7 years 3 months, are presented in Table 5.VIII. The IQ scores ranged from the low-70s in the first tests to consistently average scores on the last two occasions. Very slow language development made early test scores unreliable and invalid as predictors of intelligence potential, but they are included to provide for comparisons *between* the children. At all ages, scores fell close to the mean for the set and within the expected range of error. Such differences as there were could have been due to factors in the test situation or to fluctuations in performance. In this MZ set no child scored consistently higher or lower than any of the others and the rank order varied on each testing. Performance in the preschool years, when their language development was delayed, was well below average, but by school entry at 5 years it was firmly within the average band. Table 5.IX shows their patterns of success and failure on the subtests of the Stanford–Binet at successive testings, and illustrates quite dramatically how children of identical heredity and the same rearing environment vary in behavioural tasks.

Visual perception
Mittler (1971) considered that genetic factors play a more important role in the development of visuo-spatial abilities than in other traits commonly measured. His review of studies of laboratory-type tasks of visual perception carried out between 1960 and 1970 showed that, in comparison with DZ twins, MZ twins showed a much greater similarity of response on visual perception tests (after-image, eidetic imagery, critical flicker fusion, autokinetic phenomenon), suggesting some genetic basis for these responses (see also Anastasi 1979).

The MZ Auckland quads produced very different responses to the Stanford–Binet Draw-a-Circle item at 3 years (Fig. 5.4) and to the Frostig Copy-a-Drawing item at 7 years (Fig. 5.5), implying variations in learning and performance.

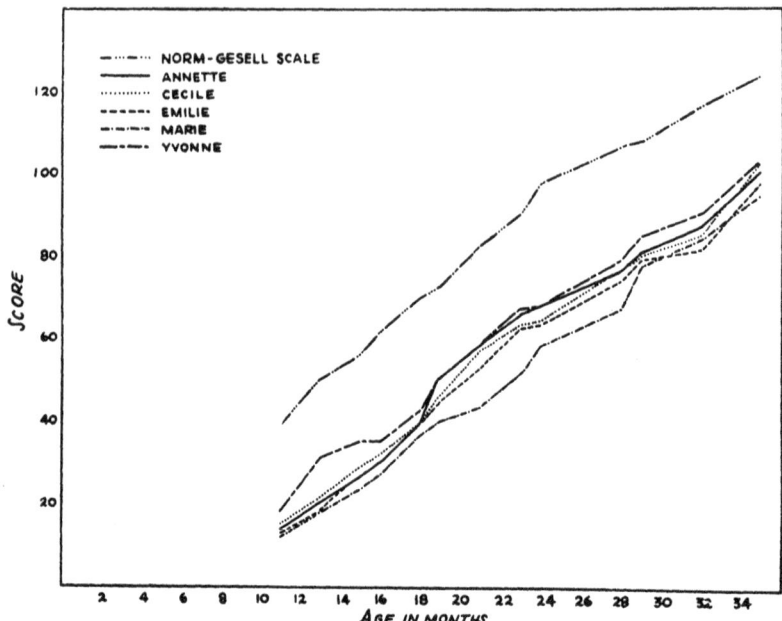

Fig. 5.2. Gesell 'developmental quotient' scores of the Dionne quintuplets between the ages of 11 months and 35 months (Blatz and Millichamp 1937).

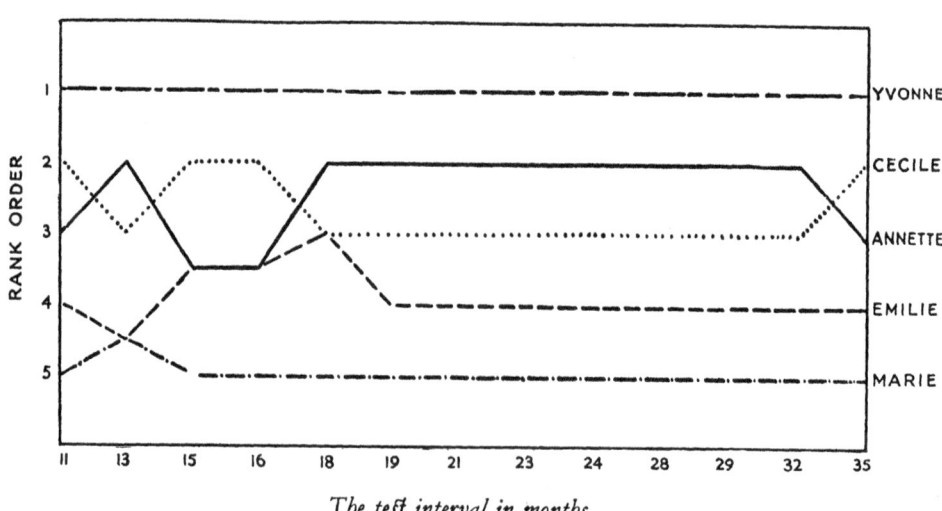

The test interval in months

Fig. 5.3. Changes in rank order of the total scores on tests of mental development for the Dionne quintuplets between the ages of 11 months and 35 months (Blatz 1939).

TABLE 5.VII
Results of intelligence tests for two sets of quadruplets

Test		GENAIN (MZ) at 10:3 yrs.*				SCHENSE (QZ) at 9:7 yrs.**			
		1	2	3	4	Joan	Jean	James	Jay
Stanford–Binet (Form L) (Terman and Merrill 1937)	MA	11:4	11:0	11:3	10:5	11:0	10:2	10:4	11:2
	IQ	110	107	109	101	115	106	107	116
Army Beta (Yoakum and Yerkes 1920)	MA	9:2	9:2	9:2	9:0	12:10	11:0	12:0	12:0
	IQ	90	90	90	87	134	115	126	126

*Bayley 1963; **Gardner and Newman 1944.

TABLE 5.VIII
Intelligence test scores and ranks for the MZ Auckland quadruplets (A, B, C, D)

Age (yrs:mths)	Test	Score				Rank			
		A	B	C	D	A	B	C	D
3:1	Stanford–Binet*	76	72	69	79	2	3	4	1
3:8	Stanford–Binet*	81	85	90	85	4	2=	1	2=
4:2	Stanford–Binet*	80	87	83	87	4	1=	3	1=
5:0	Stanford–Binet*	103	103	99	93	1=	1=	3	4
6:0	WISC**	99	104	99	100	3=	1	3=	2
7:3	Young***	107	111	108	109	4	1	3	2

*Terman and Merrill (1960); **Wechsler (1949); ***Young (1973).

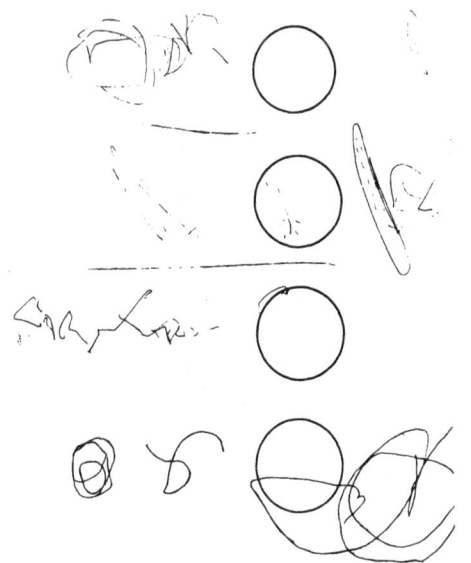

Fig. 5.4. Responses of the MZ Auckland quads at age 3 years to the 'Draw-a-Circle' task of the Stanford–Binet test.

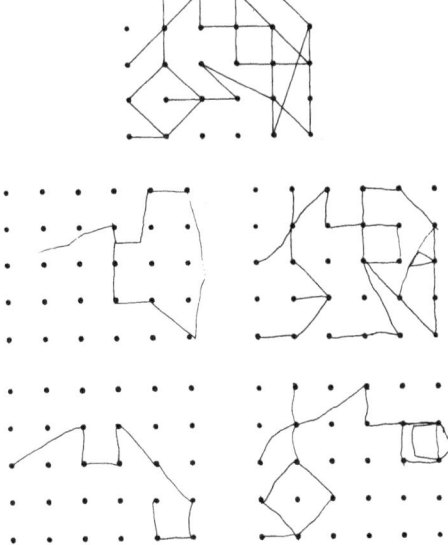

Fig. 5.5. Responses of the MZ Auckland quads at age 7 years 3 months to the Frostig 'Copy-a-Design' task.

TABLE 5.IX
Stanford–Binet subtests passed (/) and failed (0) by the MZ Auckland quadruplets at ages 3:1, 3:8, 4:2 and 5:0 years.*

Age	Subject	2:0	2:6	3:0	3:6	Age-level of test (yrs:mths) 4:0	4:6	5:0	6:0	7:0	Overall summary
3:1	A	/////	1/00/1	/0000/	000000						MA 2:6 to 2:10
	B	/////	0////	/000/0	000000						IQ 80 to 89
	C	/////	////0	1/00/0							
	D	/////	0////	/0/00/	0/0000						
3:8	A			/////	/////**	0/0/00	0----/				MA 3:4 to 3:8
	B		/////	/////	////0	/0000	0----/				IQ 92 to 100
	C		/////	//0//	////0	/0000	/----/				
	D		/////	//0//	000/1-**	//0000	0----/				
4:2	A			/////	////0	//00/0	00/000	00/0/0	000000		MA 3:10 to 4:1
	B			/////	/////	///000	0/0000	//000	000000		IQ 91 to 97
	C			/////	/////	//0//0	00/0/0	//0000	000000		
	D			/////	////0	//0/00	00/000	/0000	000000		
5:0	A							/////	0//00/	000000	MA 5:1 to 5:8
	B							/////	/0/0//	000000	IQ 102 to 112
	C					//////	0/////	00/000	000000		
	D							/////	0//0//	000000	

*The Stanford–Binet (Terman and Merrill 1960) consists of six subtests at each age-level. The test begins where a subject passes all subtests at that age-level. Quad A at age 3:1, for example, passed all six subtests for 2-year-olds, four for 2½-year-olds, two for 3-year-olds and none for 3½-year-olds. Subtests passed and failed differed from child to child. Mental age (MA) therefore varied, as did IQ, though not greatly.
**Alternative test used.

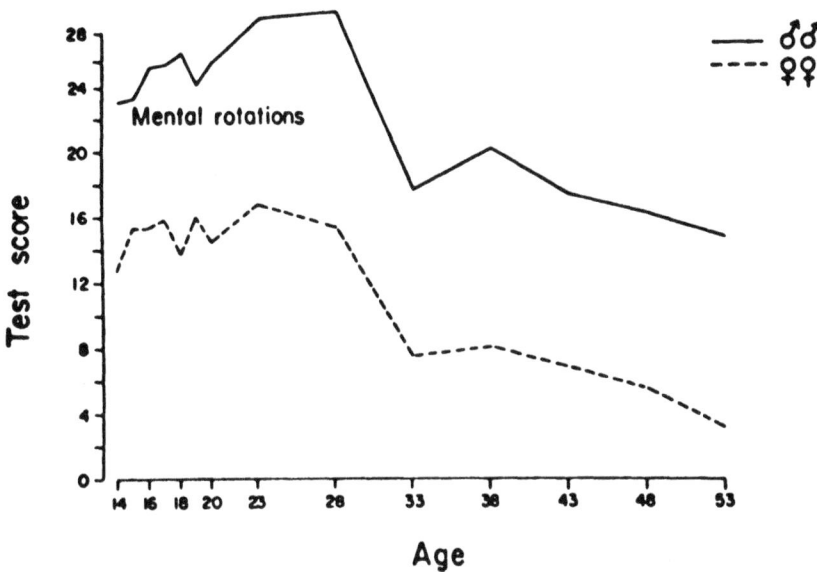

Fig. 5.6. Cross-sectional age curves for male twins and female twins on a test of spatial ability (Wilson *et al.* 1975).

Spatial ability
Consistent differences in performance on tests of spatial ability between males and females have been demonstrated. Using a Mental Rotations Test to measure this ability in 2978 twin subjects aged 14 to 53 years, Wilson *et al.* (1975) found highly significant sex and age differences, and no interaction effect (Fig. 5.6). Hypotheses to explain such consistent results have been:
★ that spatial ability is influenced by a sex-linked major gene of recessive character;
★ that it may be due to differences in hormone balance;
★ that there may be a gene for spatial ability which is both sex-linked and testosterone-limited in its expression.
Such hypotheses cannot be related to the higher perceptual or visuo-spatial scores of MZ and DZ twins reported earlier.

Spatial aspects of texts
One of the first sets of learning for the beginning reader concerns the arbitrary conventions of how books are presented. The movement possibilities as a two-handed person approaches an English book with two presented pages (left and right) are complex, and are not covered by the simple question, 'Which hand does the child prefer to use?' If the text occurs on each page, records must be kept of (i) which hand was used, (ii) to move in which direction, (iii) across which page. Figure 5.7A illustrates some behaviours which can occur when either hand is used on either page in either of two horizontal and two vertical directions. The solid arrows plot several appropriate movements using the left hand or the right hand,

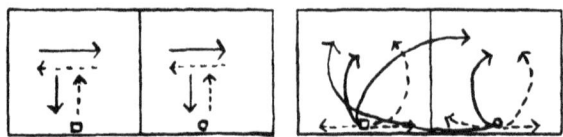

Fig. 5.7A. Hand movement possibilities when reading a book (Clay 1982).

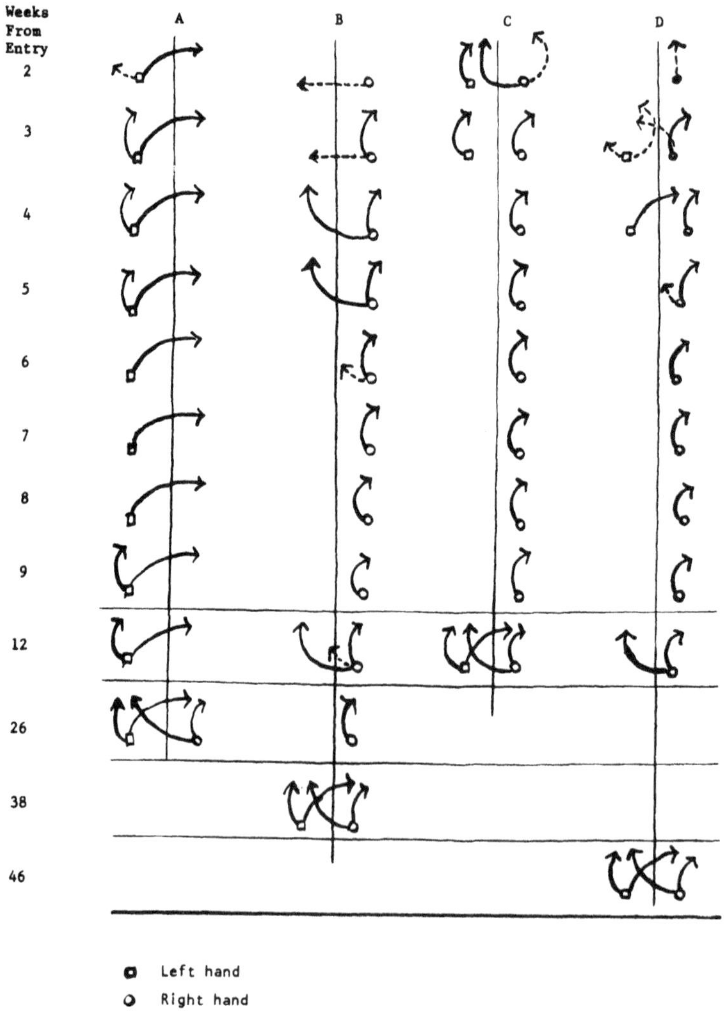

Fig. 5.7B. Reading behaviours of the MZ Auckland quads: observed hand movements in the first year of school (Clay 1982).

and the dotted arrows show a few of the inappropriate movements. Research has shown that observations close to the onset of reading instruction will detect each of these movements and others even more strange (Clay 1979).

Orientation to the spatial characteristics of texts was observed in the MZ Auckland quads at weekly intervals during their first year at school. One girl is left-handed and three are right-handed. The observed movement behaviours are illustrated in Figure 5.7B. There was a period of orienting to print in which the quads showed differences. There was another period in which an asymmetrical hand response was consistently applied. After two weeks at school one right- and one left-handed child were consistently using that preferred hand to locate their position on text. The other two took four to five weeks to establish a preferred hand. (The learning arose from the child's own choice of movements and was not tutored.) There was a later trend to optional use of either hand whatever the format of the text. In Week 12 one girl again used either hand for pointing to text, a change which gave her greater flexibility for reading text on both left and right pages. The left-hander made this move at week 26, the two others at Weeks 38 and 46 respectively. The sequence held true for the right- and the left-handed girls, and the timing of acquisition differed despite their identical heredity and similar environmental histories.

Auditory memory measured by digit recall
The ability to repeat a series of numbers is a commonly used subtest in tests of general ability. Preschool children can repeat two or three digits; 5- to 7-year-olds manage four or five. At older ages ability seems to be related to strategies for rehearsing and memorizing, and, when the subject is asked to repeat the digits in reverse order, to mental manipulations of that remembered material.

Twins T and C were trained for eight weeks in digit memory (Hilgard 1933). (As this behaviour changes slowly it was an odd ability to try to train in such a short programme.) Twin C's performance improved from two digits to three or four; twin T similarly improved to from three to five digits. After the training programme finished the performances of both twins settled to a span of three or four digits and remained at that level throughout the follow-up period. The MZ Auckland quads were particularly low scorers on digit recall tests. At 5½ years they were at the low extreme of the distribution for that age, with a span of only two digits. Their language scores showed marked retardation also, but the relationship of digit recall to language retardation probably is reciprocal.

Language development
Twins generally tend to be inferior to singletons in most measureable aspects of language acquisition. Day (1932) found that twins had smaller vocabularies, a narrower range of parts of speech, and used more immature sentences than singletons with whom they were compared. Mittler (1969, 1971) compared the performances at 4 years of 200 twins and 100 singletons on the Illinois Test of Psycholinguistic Abilities. He found the same relationships, twins showing a language delay of around six months, with low scores falling more or less equally across all subtests.

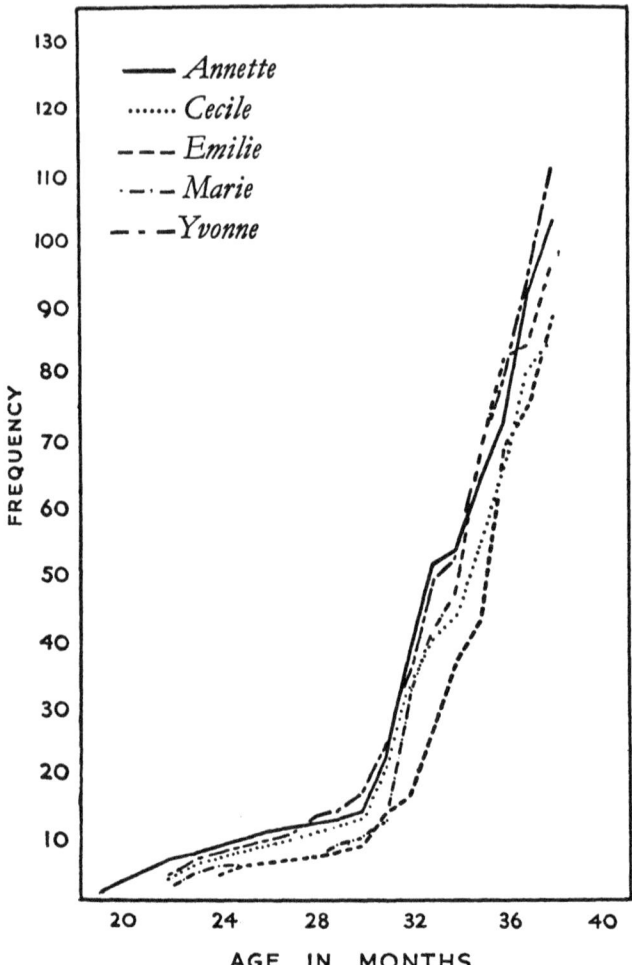

Fig. 5.8. Language development of the Dionne quintuplets: accumulative record of new words used (adapted from Blatz 1939).

A Russian set of twins, Liosha and Yura, were referred to Luria and Yudovich (1978) because of language retardation at 5 years. Two treatments were tried. Firstly a programme of language training was introduced for the twin with the poorer language (Yura), and secondly the twins were separated and placed in different kindergarten groups. Aside from small phonetic defects, Yura's vocabulary and grammar approximated the normal speech of his peers after three months, and both twins learned to use language in their play to analyse and plan constructive activity.

The Dionne quins' first language was French. Blatz *et al.* (1937a) reported that at 3½ years their speech was as much retarded when compared to that of twins as twins' speech is when compared to that of singletons. A graph plotting the number

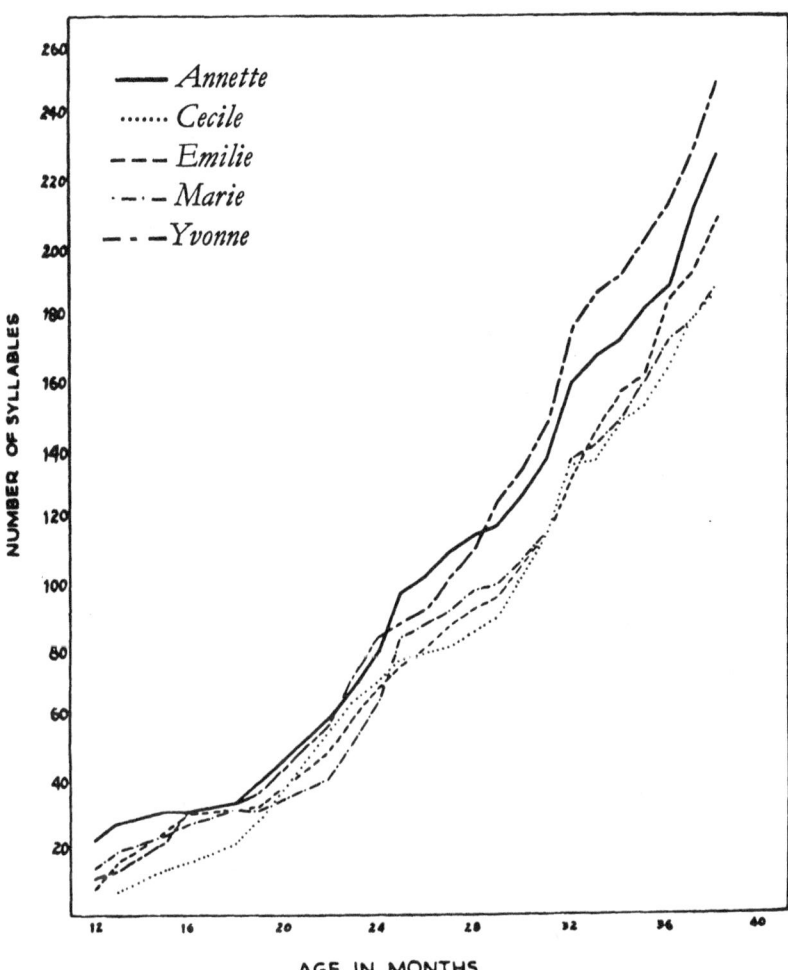

Fig. 5.9. Language development of the Dionne quins: progress in syllablization (adapted from Blatz *et al.* 1937*a*).

of new words learned (Fig. 5.8) shows a slow beginning up to 30 months and fairly steady, more rapid progress after that time. A count of syllables used yielded a different slope but showing similar progress for each child (Fig. 5.9).

When the MZ Auckland quads were first referred for developmental assessment at 2 years 9 months they had very little language and could not score on measures of language ability. This language delay received attention from a paediatrician and developmental psychologist through parent counselling, special entry to kindergarten, an individual language programme administered daily for some months before school entry and careful monitoring by the school. Despite these focused efforts, improvement was slow. At entry to school and two years later their language performance was well below average. A sentence repetition test

(Clay *et al.* 1983) for control over grammatical structures had been designed and normed on a random sample of Auckland children: the mean score for children aged between 5 and 6 years was 22 out of a possible maximum of 42. In the second week of school the quads (with scores of 3, 0, 3, 3) were between two-and-a-half and three standard deviations below that mean. The test was repeated at 7 years 3 months: although scores had improved markedly they were still only average to below-average for children aged two years younger. The Illinois Test of Psycholinguistic Abilities was also administered at 7 years 3 months; again scores were well below average for age. On both these very different measures of language ability, the rank order of the girls was the same (Table 5.X).

Summary of specific cognitive abilities
A review by DeFries *et al.* (1976) from twin and family studies failed to answer the question of whether genetically independent abilities exist. The search for a genetic base for specific abilities is confounded by the fact that we have defined cognitive abilities in terms of the tasks used to test them. Digit recall and word fluency are examples of this.

There are consistent reports of language retardation in twins. Thus it is not surprising that studies show a slight but consistent tendency—at all socio-economic levels—for twins to gain lower scores than singleton children on verbal intelligence tests. Subgroups of twins do not show consistent differences but it is possible that MZ twins are relatively more retarded than DZ twins, especially on verbal tests, and that MZ boys are more retarded than MZ girls.

Koch (1966) reported the relative inferiority of twins in quantitative, motor and spatial tests, and relative superiority in visuo-perceptual tests. This tendency is established but not explained.

DeFries *et al.* (1976) recommended large-scale adoption studies of twins to obtain unambiguous evidence of heredity as a cause of individual differences in specific cognitive abilities. Detailed behavioural studies of higher multiple sets in time series or longitudinal designs might also be a profitable approach to the study of genetic–environmental interactions. Assumptions about the relationships of test scores to genetic factors make such an alternative approach an attractive research proposition.

School progress
I have not located any published study the main focus of which was the school progress of children in multiple sets. When this topic has been reported it has often been from school reports or teacher-made tests of unknown reliability. Yet, with such poor data, behaviour geneticists and child psychologists have often used school progress as one method of estimating general intellectual ability or specific abilities. Such indicators must be recognized as unsatisfactory. An example is the report by da Silva *et al.* (1975) of the school achievement at a mean age of 12 years of 96 pairs of Brazilian twins. The authors judged their findings to be in agreement with previous conclusions of genetic determination of school achievement. MZ twins were found to be more alike in school achievement than DZ twins and this was attributed to their single-cell similarities. No consideration was given to the

TABLE 5.X

Results of language tests for the MZ Auckland quadruplets at age 7:3

Test	A	B	C	D
Illinois Test of Psycholinguistic Ability (Kirk et al. 1968)	6:2	6:8	6:5	6:3
Sentence repetition (Clay et al. 1983)*	16	23	20	19

*Average score at age 5 to 6 years = 22.

TABLE 5.XI

'General average' ability scores for the Keys quadruplets between the 3rd and 6th Grades at school*

Grade	MZ		DZ	
	Roberta	Mona	Mary	Leota
3rd	86	86	87	87
5th	95	95	89	94
6th	96	93	85	90

*Brintle (1931).

sameness of their past experience, the school's provision for them, or their mutual exchange of learning. We know almost nothing about how siblings of equal age teach each other.

The school progress of the Good quads was reported descriptively by Corner (1974):

At 5 years primary-school education began and progressed well so that all could read before 7 years . . . During the ninth year, the parents moved to a small dairy farm in a more rural area which necessitated changing the primary school. Although no serious learning problems were encountered, the children were probably understimulated, became bored with school and their education attainments fell considerably below their potential . . . Secondary education began at 11 years 3 months, in a large school where each child was placed in a different class. In the class of most able children, Bridget developed independently and achieved higher academic attainment than her sisters. She remained at school till 17 years, taking a secretarial course during her last year . . . Jennifer, Frances, and Elizabeth remained at school till 16 years, making average progress. They all learnt to play the piano and Jennifer the violin.

An early psychological report on the Keys quads (Brintle 1931) compared the MZ and DZ pairs for reading, writing, spelling, arithmetic, grammar, music and drawing between the third and sixth grades of school. Little differentiation was reflected in the 'General Average' scores that were reported (Table 5.XI).

Gesell and Thompson (1941) addressed the question as to whether there are cumulative effects of small and early achievement gains. A high achiever in a multiple set might attain and even increase the lead over his or her siblings over time. Aside from the variability of progress, assessment errors and the changing nature of tests, are such cumulative gains measureable? Can a 'compound interest'

TABLE 5.XII

Cumulative achievement measures for twins T and C between the ages of 6½ and 13 years*

Test measure	Number of tests	T ahead	C ahead	T and C equal
Oral spelling	5	1	3	1
Written spelling	6	4	2	—
Oral reading	9	5	3	1
Word test	7	7	0	—
Arithmetic	8	4	3	1
Language	4	2	1	1
Reading memory	5	0	4	1
Total	44	23	16	5

*Gesell and Thompson (1941).

concept in development be quantified? To answer these questions the authors looked at measures taken between 6½ and 13 years on twins T and C, and asked how many times twin T was ahead of twin C and vice versa. Despite the 23 to 16 tally (Table 5.XII), the authors were not prepared to say that twin T had better achievement than twin C.

From six to eight years T scored a little higher than C in all the tests given, but after this age, differences occur first in favour of one twin, then the other . . . In most individual tests now T and now C tended to excel with inconsistent fluctuations. In the reading of single words, however, T was always slightly better and in reading memories C was superior. At the age of 13 years even this consistent difference has vanished so far as test scorings indicate.

A school programme can be considered equivalent to a psychological treatment (as in an experiment), but a treatment which is unlikely to provide equivalent experiences for MZ siblings who are in different classes. Different cognitive strategies could be developed by different programmes so that word reading superiority in one sibling and higher comprehension in another might be quite consistent with programme emphases. They could also be consistent with an hypothesis of selective attention producing differences in MZ twins who were in the same programme with the same teacher.

School progress of the MZ Auckland quads: environmental effects
A detailed examination of the early progress of the MZ Auckland quads suggests that achievement can differ among MZ subjects at any one time, that rank orders on achievement measures can change from year to year and that low achievement does not necessarily yield cumulative handicaps. As no marked prenatal, birth or preschool experiences had produced differences in these children prior to school entry, would schooling itself produce any such differences?

Intelligence test scores were within the normal range and variations between the four on several testings scattered in random ways. On personal and social adjustment the girls all had similar ratings of 'passive', and family relationships were reported as very positive by each child (see pp. 42–43). On behaviours related to school progress they showed similar levels of preparation. They were all placed

TABLE 5.XIII

Timing in change of reading behaviours for the MZ Auckland quadruplets

Behaviour	Weeks from school entry to mastery			
	A	B	C	D
Directional movement				
In reading	3	3	6	26
In writing	4	2	2	4
Use of hand				
Consistently one hand	2	4	5	2
Either hand	26	12	46	38
Book language				
Gramatically acceptable sentence	12	10	4	26
Modelled on book sentence	12	10	10	26
Control over sequencing				
Word-by-word	12	12	26	46
Accuracy over 80%	38	12	46	46
Accuracy over 90%	56	38	103	—
Self-monitoring				
One self-correction in 10 errors	26	12	46	46

with the same teacher for the first year.

Weekly recording of emergent academic behaviours showed them gaining control of various reading and writing behaviours on different time schedules. At this stage of early learning the child does not read the text of a simple caption book but constructs an utterance which takes account of the story, the pictures, his or her language skills and what has been learned so far. Changes occur because the child learns to direct several sets of behaviour to the tasks of trying to read and trying to write. Table 5.XIII summarizes these changes but calls for brief explanation.

The quads were slow learners in their first year at school. At the end of 15 months (and the end of the school year) they had just completed the first book of the basic reading series. Compared with three research samples of children aged 6 years (see Clay 1985, p. 37) the quads at 6 years 3 months were in the lowest 10 per cent for that age-group (see Table 5.XV). What had they learned on what time schedule?

DIRECTIONAL BEHAVIOUR

This learning was reported earlier. Two girls (one right- and one left-handed) were weeks ahead of the other two (right-handed) girls. Flexible use of either hand for pointing to focus attention on print was reached at between 12 and 46 weeks, showing remarkably different rates of learning.

ACCURACY

Reading the first texts accurately (a 90 per cent success rate was considered satisfactory) requires the co-ordination of word-by-word locating and reading, directional behaviours, language responses and visual perception of print cues. It was in these behaviour shifts that big differences appeared in the quads' performances.

TABLE 5.XIV
Results of reading and spelling tests for the MZ Auckland quadruplets at age 7:3

	A	B	C	D
Reading age*	7:4	7:1	6:6	6:7
Spelling age	7:2	7:6	6:6	6:3

*Average of five tests.

★ Quad B attained word-by-word reading at Week 12 and took a further 26 weeks to achieve the next shift to over 90 per cent accuracy.
★ Quad A attained word-by-word reading at Week 12 but did not achieve 90 per cent accuracy until Week 56.
★ For quad C the changes came at Weeks 26 and 103.
★ For quad D the first change came at Week 46 but the second was still not completed after 115 weeks at school.

The cumulative experiences of these four children in learning to read were very different given that these observations were samples of what amounted to hundreds of attempts to read for each child throughout the year.

CONCORDANT SHIFTS

The concordance among quads A, B and C in the timings of the use of either hand for pointing to text and the shift in accuracy or self-correction which signals real reading are fascinating. The flexible use of either hand to point and the achievement of some co-ordinated control over general reading behaviours shared a temporal relationship in three of the four records. One might hypothesize that a child must learn to cross-relate visual, language and directional/spatial behaviours to become a reader, and that the acquisition of these behaviours is largely dependent on the child's interactions with his or her various environments. Genetic factors and test score similarities did not govern the time scales over which these children came to control emergent reading behaviours.

THE SECOND YEAR AT SCHOOL

Satisfactory and accelerated progress in learning to read and spell was achieved after a delayed start. Although scores on two language tests fell below the average for children 18 months younger, the retardation did not prevent progress in learning to read and spell. Reading and spelling scores improved markedly for all four subjects in the second year of school, although quads A and B showed better progress than quads C and D (Table 5.XIV).

I requested that the girls be separated into pairings each of one higher and one lower progress child, but without revealing my reasons or behavioural findings to the school. One pair went to a class of same-age or older children and the other pair to a class of same-age or younger children. Both pairs began the year at the same instructional level. Over the first half of this second year the teachers moved the two pairs on different time schedules. The pair in the class of older children moved

TABLE 5.XV

Progress through the reading book series of the MZ Auckland quadruplets in their second school year: two teaching effects*

Subject	Age-level of reading book (yrs:mths)				
	6:3		6:9		7:3
A	3	Teaching effect I	15	Teaching effect II	21
C	3		15		19
B	3		10		19
D	3		10		19

*The quads were separated into two pairs each comprising one higher and one lower progress child: A and C were placed in a class of same-age or older children, B and D in a class of same-age or younger children (teaching effect I). When the differences in progress were detected, the teaching programmes were altered accordingly (teaching effect II).

TABLE 5.XVI

Rank order of the MZ Auckland quadruplets on school attainment tests at ages 6:0, 7:3 and 12:3

Age	Test	Rank order			
		A	B	C	D
6:0	Reading	1	2	3	4
7:3	Reading	1	2	3	4
	Spelling	2	1	4	3
12:3	Listening comprehension	2	4	1*	2
	Reading comprehension	4	2	1*	3
	Reading vocabulary	3	1*	2*	4
	Mathematics	4	3	1	2

*Scores above 50th percentile for age.

more quickly through the book series than the other pair. This was clearly a teaching effect. The school's monitoring procedures detected the differences halfway through the year: the teachers changed the programme and closed the gap—a second teaching effect (Table 5.XV).

At 7 years 3 months the quads were within the average range of progress for most classroom activities. This was a success story. The retardation recorded after their first year at school had been overcome by good teaching, employing different pacing schedules in ordinary classrooms. Two teaching effects were demonstrated—one in gaining the success and the other in gaining it in different ways. These effects were not due to initial attainment differences as each pair contained a higher and a lower progress performer.

LATER ACHIEVEMENT

School progress was checked at 12 years. Results on nationally normed tests did not show any consistent cumulative advantages for the two girls who were higher achievers at 6 years and at 7 years 3 months. Intervening experiences had significantly changed the rank order of the quads on school achievement (Table 5.XVI). However, below-average achievement status did persist for all.

Personality
Researchers have from time to time turned to the study of MZ twins to answer the question, 'In what ways do either heredity or environment influence personality formation?' In general the personalities of MZ twins tend to be much alike. However, if they have been reared together then many features of their environments have also been alike. In case studies of MZ twins, differences described are often 'so slight that they would be set down as similarities if they were encountered in a study of unselected children or even of ordinary siblings' (Gesell and Thompson 1929).

Anastasi (1979) reported on personality differences in studies of older subjects. Gottesman (1963, 1965) gave the Minnesota Multiphasic Personality Index to MZ and DZ twins in Minnesota and in Boston. He obtained reasonable agreement between the two sets of data, with relatively high genetic effects for social introversion and psychopathy, and for depression and schizophrenia. Eaves and Eysenck (1975) reported that both genetic and environmental factors contributed to variation in extraversion. However, Anastasi, an authority on individual differences, defines personality measurement as an area of extreme complexity and challenge, for which no simple summary of the literature is possible.

Information from higher multiple sets
It is generally accepted that physical characteristics are affected least by environment, intelligence more, education and achievement still more, and personality the most.

Comments on higher multiple sets may report merely the interpretations of their behaviours made by adults who are trying to capture the differences among very similar children. Gardner and Newman (1943b) made the following comments on the MZ Morlok quads at 10 years:

> If we were inclined to emphasize the personality differences of this interesting group of four genetically identical individuals and to overlook their strong, fundamental resemblances, we might venture to characterize them as the "boss," the "clown," the "artist," and the "baby." Such characterizations would, however, be misleading, to say the least, for these behavior peculiarities are at best superficial and probably have arisen from slight differences in size and vigor rather than from inherent differences in personality.

The same authors found the largest differences in the five sets of quads they studied among a QZ set of two boys and two girls (the Schenses). They described the personality differences as similar to those expected in any four siblings born separately in a family (Gardner and Newman 1944).

Personality studies of the Dionne quins stressed that identical heredity with close similarity of environment does not result in identical personality, and each had in some degree a personality differing from that of the others (Blatz et al. 1937b, Scheinfeld 1952). One was a leader, dubbed 'the Matriarch', one was happy-go-lucky, another unpredictable, another more aggressive and one was 'the baby'. By 10 years of age their business manager claimed that . .

> They are absolute individualists. One is the boss of the five, another has a greater love of

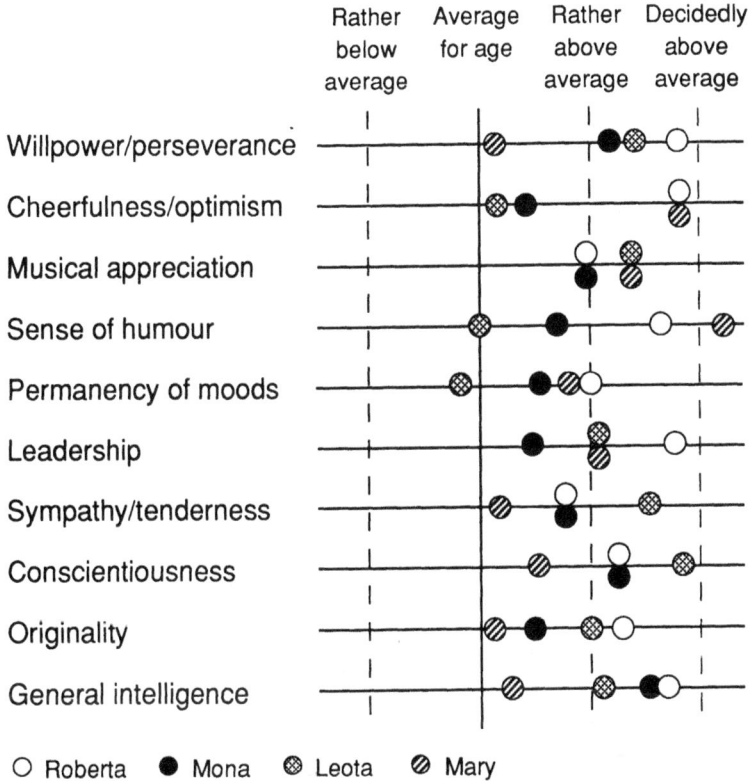

Fig. 5.10. Personality trait ratings of the Keys quadruplets at 12 years (mean ratings by four different raters) (redrawn from Brintle 1931).

clothes than the others, one is the comedienne, another the student and musician, and one the wistful, affectionate 'little sister'. (Berton 1977)

In trying to discriminate between the look-alike MZ Auckland quads I used to find myself searching for the outgoing one or the independent one. After visits at regular intervals I came to recognize that on any one day I was probably sampling a mood or response in one child that was part of a common repertoire and might appear in another member of the set on another day. Gesell and Thompson (1941) made a similar comment in regard to the twins T and C:

This virtually constant and evenly balanced companionship ... has served to keep both twins in their orbits and to stabilize their characteristics.

Most appraisals of 'personality' variables are confused with learned behaviours arising from the opportunities and pressures of being a member of a set of same-age siblings (see pp. 41–44).

One approach to personality measurement is the rating scale. Figure 5.10 shows the results at 12 years for the Keys quads, taking the average rating of four raters (Brintle 1931). The DZ pair account for every extreme measure except

TABLE 5.XVII
Results of personality assessments for the MZ Auckland quadruplets at ages 6:0, 7:3 and 12:0

Age	Test	A	B	C	D	Comments
6:0	Minnesota Adjustment Profile II*	39	37	33	33	NZ mean, 38.7
7:3	California Test of Personality**					
	Personal	20	10	10	40	Percentiles
	Social	20	10	10	40	
12:0	Round-about-twelve Self-concept***					
	Positive	22	19	24	22	32 items, maximum
	Negative	28	26	36	28	score 2 points each

*Hathaway and McKinley 1951; **Thorpe *et al.* 1953; ***Clay and Oates 1980.

leadership and general intelligence. By the age of 22 years there were marked differences in intelligence and personality between the MZ and DZ pairs, of whom the former looked very much alike while the latter differed from them and from each other.

The Minnesota Adjustment Profile II, a personality rating scale for which normative data were available for an Auckland sample of 5-year-olds, was administered to the MZ Auckland quads at 6 years. Two teachers rated each child. They considered the children similar on most characteristics and rated all four as 'passive'. Two children achieved average scores, while the other two were adjudged by the teachers to fit the description of 'quiet unforthcomingness'. At 7 years 3 months self-ratings on the California Test of Personality were obtained by reading the items with each child. Both Personal and Social Adjustment scores were below the mean for their age, ranging from the 10th to the 40th percentile. One girl, D, saw herself in a more positive light than her sisters saw themselves. At 12 years the quads completed another self-concept inventory, for which national norms were available. Individual differences were apparent, with two children deviating somewhat from the patterns of the others, one lower on positive self-concept and the other high on negative self-concept. The ratings at 6 years, 7 years 3 months and 12 years are summarized in Table 5.XVII.

Attachment

The issue of the attachment bonds that develop between parents and higher multiple sets has been raised in the literature, touching a similar area to the Family Relations Test discussed in Chapter 4 (pp. 42–43). Several factors could threaten the formation of attachment links: a tendency, reported by Spillman (1987), of some mothers of twins to reject the second twin; the separation of multiple babies for special care; exhaustion and anxiety in the mother; and most of all, the likelihood of multiple caretakers in hospital and at home. In one study of quads and quins (Krall *et al.* 1980) the Decarie measures of Object Constancy and Object Relations were obtained at three-monthly intervals up to 2 years. The authors concluded that the multiple caretaking situation in the well-educated, upper middle class, suburban families they studied did not interfere with specific attachment to the mother.

Recent reports

Three recent publications present more up-to-date approaches to developmental reports with data from tests currently in use. However, all report on multiple sets with some abnormal condition.

★ Three quintuplets with cleft palates were followed up and compared with their normal siblings at the age of 5 years (Zilberman *et al.* 1980, 1985).
★ Triplets with infantile autism were assessed for neuropaediatric status (Gillberg 1983) and with behavioural ratings and psychological tests (Burgoine and Wing 1983).
★ Several studies were undertaken on a set of 51-year-old MZ quads (the Genains), all of whom had schizophrenia (Buchsbaum *et al.* 1984, DeLisi *et al.* 1984, Mirsky *et al.* 1984—following up on earlier documentation by Rosenthal 1963). The set was of particular interest to professionals working with this psychiatric condition, and as Mirsky *et al.* reported:

> . . we have attempted to exploit virtually all the available technology in an effort to comprehend this fascinating enigma of identical quadruplets with unequal expression of schizophrenia.

It seems a pity that there are no comparable studies of quadruplets whose lives have unfolded in healthy ways.

6
PSYCHOLOGY AND HIGHER MULTIPLE BIRTHS

In this chapter the potential contribution of psychologists to the scientific study of the development of higher multiple sets will be explored, especially in relation to (i) data collection problems, and (ii) controlled studies of environments and their effects on individuality.

Twin studies have had a marked influence on the study of, and have been an important source of hypotheses about, higher multiples. Though many authors before him had collated information on multiple births, Galton (1875) gave a new twist to this scientific interest because he saw in twin studies the possibility of studying the relative contributions of heredity and environment to growth and development. He pointed to three assumptions that one might make about differences which occur between MZ twins:

★ a lack of difference would indicate a continuing genetic effect;
★ a difference could indicate a delayed or emergent genetic effect;
★ an environmental effect would be shown if one twin developed an illness and the other did not, so that differences that developed between them could be attributed to the illness.

Since that time research has compared MZ twins raised together and apart, and MZ twins with DZ twins. Twins have also been compared with various other groups like siblings and parents, and control groups of singletons. As twins live through precisely the same period of historical time, it was assumed that their similar life experiences would affect their psychological characteristics to similar extents and in similar ways, allowing some measure of control over environments. The genetic duplication in MZ subjects was thought to establish control over heredity.

Rife (1938) claimed that the ideal experiment for determining the relative importance of heredity and environment requires four types of conditions: (1) identical heredities, or (2) completely different heredities; and (3) identical environments, or (4) completely different environments. He concluded that, as only the first condition was attainable, the MZ twinning process does not lead to a clear-cut methodology for the study of heredity and environment.

Some methodological issues

In discussion of idiographic and nomothetic emphases in psychological theory and methodology, Marceil (1977) outlined a matrix of emphases which he explained with examples (Table 6.I):

A_x — could be illustrated from factor analysis which produces a peculiar hash of the characteristics of all participants;

TABLE 6.I
Marceil's matrix of idiographic and nomothetic approaches*

Method assumptions	Theoretical assumptions	
	x—Man is more alike	y—Man is more unique
A—Selective examination of many subjects	A_x	A_y
B—Intensive examination of few subjects	B_x	B_y

*Marceil (1977).

A_y — is shown on the objective personality test designed to make people appear alike, but revealing that they are unique;

B_x — would be found when we find a reliable relationship with one subject and see whether this holds from subject to subject;

B_y — would be found in studies of the individual as a self-contained universe.

Individual case studies

It is important to document the development of such low-incidence sets as quads and quins by case studies. Collating cases from the literature could lead to new insights and new questions not available to psychologists working with only one or two sets. The problem here is that the specific experiments carried out within such case studies would depend on the questions of interest to a particular researcher. It is therefore impossible to outline a standard set of psychological variables which should be included in such studies. Much of the data needed for individual case studies is also relevant to planned research on larger numbers of higher multiple births. As this is given in detail later in this chapter only a brief outline is provided here. Data to be collected should include the following.

★ Prenatal data, with particular attention to atypical histories.
★ Date and place of birth, with birth order.
★ Zygosity details in full (see pp. 32–34).
★ Physical growth data.
★ Intelligence measures on individual tests or developmental schedules. A longitudinal perspective corrects for the error of a single sampling of performance, and captures consistencies despite temporary differences at particular points in development.

In addition, a measure of environmental similarity would be valuable—there are no satisfactory precedents in the literature. This measure should attempt to capture qualitatively or quantitatively the extent to which the group have had closely similar or deliberately planned dissimilar opportunities for learning from their environments. Care should be taken that factors contributing to this measure are independent of any research variable. For example, if mother–child conversation is the object of study then an environmental similarity measure should not include overlapping topics like (i) Do they spend a lot of time all together with any one member of the family? or (ii) Do family members address them as a group or engage in conversation with them individually?

Methods of twin study
The kinds of questions a psychologist might want to ask about a higher multiple birth are almost infinite in scope. The single set is unlikely to contribute answers to the questions raised about heredity issues. The particular advantages to be borne in mind in the study of a single set stem from the control over environmental factors that may be available. While the methodologies of twin study do not provide immediately satisfactory research models for the study of higher multiples, they are informative and have some relevance (i) for the analysis of members of a set by twinning (*i.e.* grouping in all the available pairs), (ii) for comparison of MZ and DZ subgroups within a set, and (iii) for comparison of sex subgroups within a set.

In 1972 Gedda (Director of the Gregor Mendel Institute of Medical Genetics and Twin Research, Rome) outlined the clinical methods that have been used in the study and reporting of atypical patterns of development, disease or psychiatric conditions in one or both of a pair of (usually MZ) twins. Four types of cases may be found, as follows.
(1) Both twins are affected in the same environment. Each twin has the value of a statistical universe to be compared with the other. Comparison can be made of the changes in rapidly evolving systems or characteristics, and questions answered about organic treatment or historical time effects.
(2) One of an MZ set of twins is affected when both are in the same environment. This is a unique opportunity for study. When one twin is affected by endogenous disease the researcher can study what amounts to the same individual at the same time in good health and in illness.
(3) Both of MZ twins are affected in different environments. This is the classic case of hereditary diseases and provides a valuable opportunity to recognize their genetic nature.
(4) Only one of MZ twins is affected in different environments. If the hereditary nature of the disease can be shown, this case is very useful for studying the influence of environment on the penetrance and expression of the disease.

Gedda (1963) discussed the possible statistical significance of a single MZ twin case concordant for a given disease. This would depend upon (i) confirmation of zygosity, (ii) evidence for the partly or entirely hereditary aetiology of the case, and (iii) specific exclusion of phenocopies. An MZ pair could be considered as a statistical universe, not a statistical unit, he claimed. His argument depends on the assumption that a certain number of symptoms cannot occur by chance in both members of a pair: such coincidence must have a cause which would lie in the twins' genotype. His logic applies to the study of genetic effects of known aetiology and could only provide weak evidence for environmental effects by negating the genetic hypotheses.

Twin control experiments
Early this century twins were used in an experiment addressing a question about environmental effects. One member of a pair of twins was kept lying on his side most of the time while the co-twin was kept lying on his back in order to test the effects of these positions on the infants' head shapes (Walcher 1905, Elsässer 1906—reviewed by Price 1950). In a later application of the procedure the effects of

thiamine supplements on growth, vision and learning were studied with a large number of MZ pairs. In the psychological literature the work of Gesell and his students on twins T and C is known for its contested conclusions about the importance of maturation in the timing of emergent behaviours like walking and stair-climbing. Such experiments are referred to as twin control experiments or co-twin control studies.

Twin control studies are used to compare the merits of one medical treatment or learning programme with another. The procedure does not involve assumptions about the origin of the medical, psychological or other function with which it may be dealing, and it is not therefore significantly affected by the prenatal and natal biases outlined by Price (1950). Allowance can be made for any existing intrapair differences in initial scores, although the interaction of such differences with final scores should be considered (that is, a difference may indicate two stages or states which interact differentially with the treatment or learning opportunity). This approach is fully experimental as the researcher knows the circumstances at the start of the experiment and what goes into it.

Twin control experiments should involve the deliberate selection of the most similar MZ pairs available. An essential part of the method is measurement of the status of each individual twin before the start of the experiment. By excluding the least similar one-third or half of the available sample, the monochorial (MC) twins who usually show greater differences will tend to be omitted. This would be efficient testing procedure for co-twin work. If tests are to be conducted over a long period of time with sets of multiples it might be wise to select only dichorionic (DC) MZ pairs since latent effects of prenatal factors might show up in MC-MZ twins after the longitudinal study is underway. This would be more critical if only a small number of pairs were used, and the problem would be reduced where a larger group was used.

What are the implications of such comments for the study of higher multiples? MZ sibs present a measure of control over the genetic factors, and the day-to-day life experiences and child-rearing patterns. The danger to validity of results in this case is contamination of the effects of training (in a psychological experiment) because of cross-fertilization of responses or ideas. The children may show each other what they have learned. This is not a hazard for research design in a medical treatment with drugs when placebos are used. However, a placebo-like situation in a psychological experiment has to be designed with care. Cross-fertilization of learned responses in a psychological experiment is problematic, and with higher multiples may be impossible to avoid.

Two studies by Plomin and Willerman (1975) of reflection–impulsivity in children should be mentioned here because the report combined the two approaches to twin study reviewed so far in order to get a better check on (i) genetic factors, and (ii) their modifiability. One of these studies, involving 54 pairs of MZ twins, had suggested that reflection–impulsivity could be influenced by genetic factors. To examine the modifiability of the trait, Plomin and Willerman also set up a co-twin control study with three pairs of 4-year-old MZ twins. A double cross-over design was used. One twin in each pair was trained in impulse control for three weeks, while the co-twin was trained in verbal fluency. After three weeks the training of the twins was switched. Behaviours were assessed at three intervals, pre-training, mid-training and post-training. After a total of 18 hours training, reflection–impulsivity was not modified. It is not the point of this review to discuss whether that result could have been due to the design of the experiment, the training schedules or the tasks used, but rather to point to the innovative use of the dual approach to a genetic–environmental interaction. Note that close study of the modifiability of behaviour necessitates a drastic reduction of numbers of subjects, which applies whether the design takes the form of pre-test, training, post-test or time series designs (see below). The authors emphasized that, had they reported the results of only one of their pairs, it might have been concluded that impulse control training was effective, and they cautioned against working with single pairs.

Plomin and Willerman argued that co-twin control studies provide an estimate of the power of environmental manipulations to change behaviour. The few studies available in the literature fall into three groups: (1) attempts to demonstrate that maturation interacts with training (Gesell and Thompson 1929, Strayer 1930, Hilgard 1933, Fowler 1965); (2) comparisons of the effectiveness of different training programmes (Vandenberg 1968, on a study by Naeslund); (3) studies of the extent to which environment can produce differences in genetically identical individuals (Mirenva 1935, Vandenberg et al. 1968, Clay 1982).

The method provides a unique opportunity to control genetic variability in certain kinds of research with children, especially when (i) the time requirements of an experimental procedure preclude the use of large numbers of subjects, (ii) genetic variability is so great that it reduces the likelihood of detecting small but true differences or contributes to the failure to replicate such differences, or (iii) the degree of control it allows is needed in order to verify results obtained by experimental studies using large numbers of subjects in less intensive situations and yielding slight but significant differences.

Zygosity in the Plomin and Willerman study was determined by questionnaire on physical similarity: other researchers would need to establish their samples on a better basis than that before investing intensive effort in a time-consuming training programme. However, presumably the selection of four pairs for training could have been done on the basis of the most similar MZ pairs. An implication for the potential use of quadruplets is that genetic hypotheses derived from large-scale twin studies might be subjected to intensive tests of modifiability in a larger multiple set. In particular the use of an MZ-DZ quadruplet set would be interesting.

Twin control treatment programmes
Unsatisfactory statements can be found even in recent literature on the use of MZ twins to sort out issues concerning teaching methods. Edwards (1968), reporting to medical readers, asked:

> Have twins any future as a source of increasing knowledge by research, particularly in relation to the opportunities available in obstetrics? I will not consider their value in education or psychiatry, as this does not appear to be in doubt: for example, *the value of the new alphabet, the new maths* or of physical methods of treating psychoses *could easily be*

demonstrated on a small number of identical twins: alternative methods of demonstration have already been both expensive and uninformative. [My italics.]

More recently, Jarvik (1975) made this recommendation to psychologists:

. . a more productive approach might be to set definite goals, for example, to teach children of a given age to read with a predetermined level of proficiency after a predetermined period of instruction. There should be no difficulty in accurately, reliably, and validly measuring the preinstructional and postinstructional reading levels and in equating reasonably well the type of instruction administered. It should be possible to get several groups composed of monozygotic twin pairs, each group being homogeneous for the level and patterns of intellectual functioning, as measured by factor scores or otherwise. Different teaching methods could then be applied to the two halves of each group, each half being composed of one of the two co-twins. It should not take too long to determine in that way which method of instruction appears to be best suited for which level and pattern of intellectual functioning.

Such an experimental design has three advantages: (1) Twins are readily available, and (2) the studies could, therefore, be carried out at minimal expense, and (3) such studies would be entirely ethical since there is no clear-cut evidence at this time in favor of one teaching method over any other.

As a researcher in the acquisition of reading and writing behaviours, I am amazed at the naivety of these statements. Theorists do not agree on what reading behaviour consists of. It cannot be measured reliably for the first year or two of instruction by the usual test instruments. It is not clear what different methods consist of. It is very difficult to mount two adequately distinct teaching programmes for teaching reading because teachers will change all manner of other variables such as time spent, or use of reading in other periods. Parents and home experiences do contribute to the differences in children's progress. Method of instruction might be more related to temperament (teacher's or child's) than to levels of intellectual functioning. And outcomes may not be a matter of linear, quantitative gains, but rather of how a host of information processing behaviours become organized and available for subsequent learning. The data I have reported on the MZ Auckland quadruplets illustrate differences in their progress on many of the underlying performances needed in reading (see pp. 62–63). Theirs was a story of differential progress under the same instruction programme. There is little point in wasting the natural experimental control provided by MZ multiples on naive psychological hypotheses that do not reflect the current state of knowledge.

In a study of early reading in preschool children, Fowler (1965) gave reading instruction to five children using their co-twins as his untutored control group. The subjects were three sets of black MZ twins, and one set of white DZ triplets (MZ_1, MZ_2, DZ). MZ status was established by sound procedures, serological tests yielding perfect correlations. The twin who had the lowest IQ in each pair (including the MZ triplet pair), plus the DZ triplet, were placed in the experimental group, and tutoring was conducted for 15 to 20 minutes, four to five days per week over a period of several months, using both group and individual teaching. The span of the programme varied from two-and-a-half to five months according to the ability of the children to learn. None of the control group showed any indication of ability to read words, letters or sentences either before or after the reading programme. Of the five tutored children, two became fluent readers of text-type material, while the other three made some progress in identifying word and letter units although none reached a point of reading whole sentence units independently. The demonstration was not noteworthy, but its use of twins and triplets was insightful and in a more tightly controlled study, where treatments were more operationally defined and effects frequently measured, it could be a workable approach.

A variation would be to provide the same treatment for each twin group except in one respect, *e.g.* amount of time spent, or with or without writing, or with or without simple story books. That would provide a standard situation in that each twin faces a similar novel learning situation and tries to respond to the task's demands, but one twin has supplementary experience. Such an approach would allow better use of the triplet situation. Fowler was not able to make use of a three-way comparison because one of the MZ twins within the set was taught to read but the co-twin was not; thus, in this instance the MZ–DZ contrast was not revealing. If all the triplets had learned to read by the same approach but one MZ triplet had had supplementary experience, then a three-way comparison of MZ_1 with MZ_2, MZ_1 with DZ, and MZ_2 with DZ might have provided a demonstration of environmental effect creating differences between the MZ pair and similarity between the MZ_2-DZ pair.

The interactions of genetics and early environments are very resistant to separation for the purposes of research control when later learning is studied. A well-designed experiment with preschool multiple sibs may be unable to uncover the effects of training because of differences which began in the various environments of the uterus.

Study of a large sample of triplets
Miettinen (1954) reported a study of 633 sets of twins born in Finland between 1902 and 1952. In a follow-up study (Miettinen and Grönroos 1965), information was reported on 76 complete sets of triplets. Three sets were MZ (one male, two female), 35 sets were DZ and 38 sets were TZ. Only 15 sets came from towns and the remainder came from rural districts. Three notable features of this study are: (i) it was a follow-up study of higher multiples; (ii) the sample was large; (iii) zygosity was established to a high level of probability. Miettinen personally examined all the triplets in their homes. For most triplet sets, examinations took place at the same time so that comparisons were easy and reliable. Particular physical measurements were taken following a general physical examination. The study reported the sex distribution, growth and physical development, handedness, mental development and morbidity.

From the present author's point of view as a psychologist there were some unsatisfactory aspects of this study.
★ Information about delivery, birthweight, deformities and medical history was provided at interview by the parents, older siblings or the triplets themselves.
★ Mental development was *estimated* from the medical and historical data about learning to walk and talk, from school attendance and reports, from parental occupation, and from performance during an individual three-hour examination. No intelligence tests were given.

Using physical growth data the study provided an example of analysis by twin pairs. The triplets were divided into three pairs (A/B, A/C, B/C). In this way, the MZ triplets each provided three MZ pairs; the DZ triplets, one MZ and two DZ pairs; and the TZ sets, three DZ pairs: a total of 226 twin pairs. This total comprised 44 MZ pairs, 102 same-sex DZ pairs and 80 mixed-sex DZ pairs. MZ triplets and the MZ pairs within DZ triplet sets differed from each other in physical measurements much less than did same-sex DZ pairs in both DZ and TZ triplet sets. In general, the triplets did not seem to lag behind other Finnish children of comparable age in terms of height, even though 70 per cent were born preterm.

Such a large-scale study of subjects of different ages, at widely dispersed locations and across large spans of historical time will only rarely be undertaken.

Within-subjects designs with single subjects
Twin control studies have some features in common with more recent developments in single-subject research designs. Careful monitoring of changes in individuals as a result of treatments are a feature of both approaches. However, the early studies reported influences which minimized environmental effects; the recent developments in single-subject designs attend to environmental variables which are functional in producing changes. Strictly speaking, the research designs used with a multiple set would usually be time series designs (see below) but single-subject designs will be discussed first. They may have applications to the study of single members of multizygotic sets.

SINGLE-SUBJECT DESIGNS
Single-subject designs are quasi-experimental time series analyses (Campbell and Stanley 1963, Hersen and Barlow 1976, Kratochwill 1978). They have been widely used in behaviour analysis research with children. The emphasis is placed on the individual subject, who is exposed to two or more conditions in successive time periods. Applied to the study of a higher multiple set, this would mean that four or more individual analyses are made, and similarities and differences in timing or level of response are examined. A treatment could show differential patterns of response from individual members of the set over a similar baseline pattern.

Reversal designs. In a time series analysis the behaviour of interest is measured frequently over time. One can analyse the trend of the data as well as the magnitude of the effect. The change that is recorded may be due to a variety of factors. To increase confidence that a functional relationship exists between a variable and a change in trend it is necessary first to establish a baseline (A) as a basis of forecasting what the level of behaviour will be in future. The variable conditions (B) are then introduced, and finally baseline conditions (A) are reverted to. The reversal design has major drawbacks. Some behaviour changes are not reversible. Once you have successfully taught a particular concept there is no way to reverse the student's history and a reversal may be politically or ethically unwise. A manipulation may be so aversive that a return to the original condition occurs almost immediately. Or one may start with some unwanted response, go to a preferred response and not wish to return to the original behaviour.

Multiple baseline designs with single subjects. One variant of this design enables two or more behaviours of the same subject to be measured at the same time. After initial baseline measures are obtained on both, the experimental manipulation is applied to only one behaviour. The change obtained is compared with the level forecast for that behaviour from its baseline. The comparison of interest is between baseline (pre-training) and treatment (post-training), not between sets of behaviours. The remaining behaviours serve to support the baseline forecast of the first behaviour.

These experimental designs are frequently useful in natural or field settings. Where the experimenter has no real control over the application of the intervention, as in real-life situations such as family settings, s/he can systematically record observations before and after the intervention.

TIME SERIES DESIGNS WITH MORE THAN ONE SUBJECT

Elementary time series. In this design the dependent variable is observed over time. At some point in this observational sequence an intervention occurs with expectation of a change in the dependent variable. The nature of this intervention effect should be predicted before the analysis can begin. The causal inference depends on determining if an intervention occurring in the midst of the observational sequence has interrupted or changed the time series. From study to study the designs will differ because of the way in which the intervention is applied over time and across time.

Interrupted time series. A single intervention may be applied close to the middle of a sequence of observations across a large number of cases. The causal inference is based on discovering an abrupt change in the values taken by the dependent variable, a change in level or scope, or both.

Equivalent time series. Any extraneous event that happens to occur at the same time as the intervention can provide a threat to the internal validity of the interrupted time series design because of its lack of control for history. One way of controlling for this is to apply the intervention at several distinct points of time. Only an unusual sequence of coincidence could then yield the historical explanation.

When it is not ethically or practically feasible to assign students randomly to experimental or control groups in order to verify the effect of a life experience or treatment intervention, one of the time series designs discussed above, of sufficient length, uses the subjects as their own controls.

Multiple time series designs. These have particular application to the study of children from multiple sets. The individual members with equivalent (or similar) baseline behaviours are successively exposed to a treatment. For example, in the study of quads, Q_1 may be introduced to treatment (*e.g.* entry to a language programme) after two weeks baseline study, while Q_2, Q_3 and Q_4 remain in the baseline conditions with measures continuing to be taken. Then successively at Weeks 4, 6 and 8 these subjects are also moved one by one into the treatment. A successive change in trend for each subject coinciding with the introduction of treatment contributes to the confidence with which the changes can be linked to the treatment. Individual differences in the slope of the trend and the level may occur. If an historical event is responsible for some effects then both control and experimental time series should display the same interruption.

Because the internal validity of this design rests upon the equivalence of the control and experimental groups, the pretest measures are important, zygosity status may be critical, and assignment to treatment should usually be random. A major threat to the causal inference is cross-contamination of the control group by the experimental group. Usually steps would be taken to isolate the experimental and control groups to prevent such contamination effects. This may be very difficult with quadruplet or higher multiple sets.

Advantages claimed for these designs over the single-subject designs would apply to studies of multiple sets.

★ Statistical analyses of a more traditional kind can be used.
★ The several cases may be studied over shorter periods of time than in single-subject designs.
★ It is possible to evaluate the actual functional form of the effect, *i.e.* whether a given intervention alters the slope, the intercept or both, and this information may be important for theoretical or practical implications.
★ It is more practical when large numbers of longitudinal measurements are not possible.

Close and detailed recording in well-designed studies of responses to environmental treatments could be used to compare the learning of higher multiples under different treatments, the stability of the acquired behaviour and the tendencies of such behaviours to drift back to a similar level of performance once treatment is discontinued. Single-subject research designs have reached a high level of sophistication, and control and statistical procedures have been applied to the analysis of the changes that occur. The approach lends itself well to interventions that are helpful, such as adding some learning to the subject's repertoire or changing some unwanted behaviour for a more desired one, at the same time as the functional relationships between the changes and the treatment introduced are being studied.

An A-B-A design applied to twins

An example of experimental control over the treatment of one twin pair was made by Cunningham and Barkley (1978). 5½-year-old MZ male twins of low-normal intelligence were referred to a paediatrician for evaluation of a drug treatment they were receiving for hyperactivity. Their scores on an activity rating scale and a parent symptom questionnaire placed these boys more than three standard deviations above the mean for children of their age.

The research design was called a triple-blind, within-subject, drug–placebo, single-case reversal design, with each subject serving as his own control.

★ There was a baseline period (A), during which neither child received medication or placebo tablets.
★ In Period 2, Subject 1 received drug B; Subject 2 received placebo A_1.

★ In Period 3, Subject 1 received placebo A_1; Subject 2 received drug B.
★ In Period 4, Subject 1 received drug B; Subject 2 received placebo A_1.

These two designs may be summarized as $A\text{-}B\text{-}A_1\text{-}B$ and $A\text{-}A_1\text{-}B\text{-}A_1$ respectively. Before the first session a staff paediatrician randomly assigned the children to the individual sequences, and placed medication and placebo tablets in a series of dated envelopes. The parents, children and experimenters therefore were blind to the various drug and placebo conditions.

The boys were observed in a standard room in set task situations, interacting with their mother, and at free play for 15 minutes each during each of the experimental periods, and the behaviour was coded for 60 behavioural sequences in each 15 minute period. Observer reliability was checked.

There was a clear improvement in the quality of the children's social behaviour while on medication and their mother proved to be more responsive to the interactions that were initiated. There was a marked increase in compliance and sustained attention to the activities assigned during structured task situations, associated with an increase in the frequency with which the mother rewarded, or attended to, compliant behaviour.

Planned research with higher multiples
Locating subjects

If child psychologists have to rely on finding a report in the medical literature for prenatal, birth and neonatal information, two major sources of bias arise because (i) there has to be a medical reason for a paper to be published in a medical journal, and since the preparation for and care of higher multiple births is now well documented, fewer reports of healthy uncomplicated deliveries may be published, and (ii) there is a tendency not to report multiple births where some of the babies died or had malformations.

Birth and infancy reports appear in two places: medical journals and the press. Sometimes the authors of the journal articles will have maintained contact with the families; usually they have not. Occasionally a paediatrician has followed through to a full developmental report, or an author of a birth report has written for details to a paediatrician later in the children's development. To date the *New York Times Index* has been a source for the announcement of the birth and of early survival over a month or two. Subsequent mentions depend on the whim of a reporter going back to reports of previous sets when a new set hits the news. Such citations become inbred: the press libraries hold the news they have selected to report in the past. And as noted in Chapter 1, it is an inevitable result of public interest and press pressure that families and their medical advisers often deliberately make it difficult for attention to be directed to such children.

Two other (untested) ideas for the location of sets of multiples are available. Twin clubs, first formed in the 1930s, have become a common source of support for mothers of twins (see Appendix 2). Mothers of higher multiples could sometimes be located through this source. On the other hand, guidance may be sought by the children's parents or schools from school psychologists, or paediatricians may call for psychological checks on healthy development to be made. The local association of psychologists may provide a way of locating multiple sets.

National birth statistics and, in many countries, twin registers may provide useful information sources. Again, it must be stressed that ethical standards should be strenuously applied, and individual rights and privacy respected, in all case-finding exercises.

Prenatal and birth records and zygosity determination
When Price (1950) reviewed the primary biases of twin studies and explored (i) the natal effects, (ii) the lateral inversion effects, and (iii) the effects of mutual circulation in twins, he pointed out an important research design problem. Even if these were the only effects a researcher wished to control, s/he could not achieve such control because there are three kinds of biasing factors and only two kinds of twins.

Despite the long history of discussion concerning the natal factors, Price argued that the information we have about them today is no more convincing than that which was available a century or more ago, and will remain so until or unless the problem is approached systematically (see below). This does not mean collecting physicians' opinions after multiple births have occurred. It means obtaining their co-operation in advance so that they can commence record-keeping with suspected multiple confinements, and thus secure data that are comparable from case to case on crowding, position *in utero* and all important circumstances of delivery. Cases would need to be followed until zygosity could be determined before vital decisions to include them in a research project could be made.

After critically reviewing published accounts of quintuplet and higher order conceptions, Cameron *et al.* (1969) made recommendations for proper examination of the placenta and adequate genotyping in multiple pregnancies. In their opinion, such examinations should include:
★ the appropriate identification and labelling at birth of the babies and the portions of the cords remaining attached to the placenta;
★ the obtaining of labelled samples of blood from each cord;
★ the examination of the fresh placenta so that (i) the number and identity of the chorionic sacs is determined, (ii) samples are taken for enzyme examination, (iii) a *fetus papyraceus* is not missed, and (iv) other features, not immediately relevant to zygosity determination but relevant to fetal growth, are assessed.

It is worth reiterating that the essentials of zygosity determination (see pp. 32–34) are an accurate description of placentation, with detailed blood grouping, or the use of the minisatellite DNA probe on blood or placental tissue. The two latter methods may only be available in a specialist laboratory.

Van den Daele (1974) provided a listing of natal and prenatal factors to be considered. He assumed that the physical environment during pregnancy, parturition and the immediate neonatal period consists of factors which are known to interact with genetic factors. In addition to sex and age factors, his list is grouped under four major headings: (i) prenatal organismic, (ii) prenatal environmental, (iii) perinatal organismic, and (iv) perinatal environmental.

Using 12 sets of MZ twins aged between 24 and 90 months, van den Daele tested a large number of pre- and perinatal factors and their relationship to intelligence scores. He found no relationship between within-pair differences in intelligence and specific perinatal factors (position of presentation, use of forceps, neonatal Apgar score, birth order, birthweight). The only factors significantly correlated with intelligence (in a negative direction) were exposure to ionizing radiation during pregnancy and neonatal maturity.

Design issues and the interpretation of findings
Opposing world views
The nature–nurture issue has been argued from opposing world views. Within the Newtonian mechanical world view a complex event is analysed into more and more simple parts until the ultimate static substance is found. The simple components are then inter-related in a unidirectional and linear causal sequence (see Overton 1973).

A different world view emerges if activity rather than static properties is taken as primary. If events are constantly changing and coming into being, then the first research step may be the discovery of a system or organization within which such change occurs. There is reciprocal causality or interaction in the subsystems of this total system. There are no completely independent efficient causes*: they trigger, enhance or dampen reciprocal processes. At its logical extreme this view would hold that the interaction between components prevents the identification of the components themselves. Relatively short-term occurrences and traumatic events provide weak interactions which might be analysed under 'the convenient fiction that they are independent. To the extent that this fiction is considered reasonable the traditional experimental procedures and statistical techniques are appropriate' (Overton 1973). A strong interaction would arise from the continual reciprocity between genetic and environmental activity occurring from before conception through to the time of testing. When strong interactions appear, the traditional experimental analytic procedures become inappropriate and different types of questions need to be asked.

Each world view leads to its own scientific paradigm, theories, methods and empirical enquiries. Each is incompatible with the other and the choice between them appears to be more a rational activity than an empirical one. Historically, twin research has been Newtonian in emphasis; behavioural geneticists are now addressing questions of interaction with new vigour (see pp. 91–92).

Generalizing to singleton populations
Can one generalize from twin or higher multiple set data to the population at large? Over 98 per cent of the human beings to whom twin research is generalized have never been exposed to the condition. Schaie (1975) argued that there are astonishingly few documented differences between twins and non-twins amounting to an average difference of little more than five IQ points and a slight increase in left-handedness. For him, twins do not seem different enough from non-twins in their general personality and ability characteristics to restrict generalization. In the case of higher multiple groups, authors have been reluctant to consider generalization; the sets have been reported as unusual or exceptional cases and,

---
*An *efficient cause* is defined as an external agent or force, or independent variable, that regularly precedes and produces a phenomenon (see Baltes *et al.* 1977, p. 25).

with the notable exception of the work of Gardner and Newman, there has been a failure to collate and codify the available information, sparse though it is.

Schaie asked whether the interpersonal environment defined by the relationships of twins to each other and of others to the pair was rather special and unusual, and a threat to generalization. This problem is magnified in higher multiple sets.

MZ multiples are not necessarily identical
There can be differences in the genetic inheritance of MZ twins from conception because of chromosome errors and there can be differences in lateral inversions with mirror-image effects resulting from cytoplasmic differences. An extensive literature exists of medical cases in which MZ twins differ in their health histories, directed toward a search for genetic influences (*e.g.* Jarvik and Falek 1961, Pearson *et al.* 1963, Potter and Taitz 1972). MZ multiples may be genetically identical but are not necessarily so. Reports of higher multiples are consistent with twin data.

Prenatal development
How similar is the prenatal development of MZ multiples? In many and complex ways the maternal–fetal interactions may determine phenotypic variation in MZ twins. The fetal environment may differ because of factors like implantation, inequalities in the supply of nutrients and fetal position *in utero*. The hazards of monochorionic placentation can lead to greater differences between twins in the intra-uterine environment for MZ sets than for DZ sets. This is reflected in the incidence of abnormality among such fetuses and in problems of mutual circulation in placentae.

Environments and MZ similarities
The assumptions that researchers make about environments in which twins develop have been questioned. In the most simple form these have supposed that environmental influences will have little effect on producing differences in twin behaviours, and differences between MZ and DZ twins raised together are usually attributed to genetic influences. Environments may produce similar effects on MZ multiples. Wilson (1934) reported MZ twins to share a more similar environment than DZ twins in nearly all cases on a variety of measures. They spent more time together, were more often dressed alike and were more likely to engage in the same activities. They would, of course, be same-sex children, which may account for some of this similarity. Wilson concluded that the *reputation of being identical* contributed to greater environmental similarity for MZ twins, so that the importance of heredity might be overstated in research studies.

Environments and MZ dissimilarities
Can the environment exaggerate differences in MZ multiples? Some researchers have suggested that intrapair rivalry and competition in MZ siblings are such that individual differences are emphasized, while Loehlin (1975) concluded that a 'contrast effect' could operate, 'in which the twins (or those around them) pick out and exaggerate whatever differences there are between the members of a pair.'

This might lead not only to differences in personality characteristics, but also to differentials in opportunities to learn from different aspects of the environment.

Environmental differences for MZ and DZ multiples
Dibble *et al.* (1978) gave a series of questions to mothers of twins concerning the confusing of twins by parents and by strangers. Mothers reported that 78 per cent of MZ twins and 10 per cent of DZ twins were confused by mother and/or father, and that 99 per cent of MZ and 16 per cent of DZ twins were confused by strangers. Such information casts doubts on the assumption of environmental equivalence in studies which compare MZ and DZ twins. If male and female twins as well as MZ and DZ twins have significantly different prenatal and postnatal experiences, the contributions of genetic and environmental factors become more difficult to assess. The interactional patterns involving sex, zygosity, parity, maternal age and other variables require complex multivariate and covariate models rather than simple MZ and DZ contrasts in twin studies. According to Dibble *et al.*, the requirement that environmental differences must be accounted for in models concerning genetic contributions may make the research design more difficult, but 'the work is also made more interesting, and the complex interactions may suggest new hypotheses for future research.'

Variables with no known genetic transmission
When studies of twins broadened in scope from variables with simple genetic control to include psychological variables like intelligence, achievement and personality, the testing of assumptions about the influence of heredity and environment moved into two further classes of difficulties. The variables were test scores purporting to represent abstract and global variables which had no known genetic transmission even of a complicated form. A genetic base could only be assumed. The problem was complicated by questions about the validity and reliability of the instruments used to produce measures of these variables. The effects of the environment seem to be least for physical growth, and progressively greater for intelligence, achievement, personality and temperament (Rife *et al.* 1938).

Henderson (1975) has pointed out that those researchers who construct good measuring instruments set out to reduce the effects of environmental fluctuations. They choose items which maximize test–retest reliability and which provide stability of measures. Data from such tests are less likely to indicate short-term environmental effects or genetic–environmental interactions in the test scores of individuals. Behavioural records rather than standardized tests may show these up more readily. Intelligence test and achievement test scores might have been appropriate for psychological studies in the 1930s and 1940s, but they are used today to the neglect of more detailed, analytic and controlled techniques developed since that time for the study of behaviour and behaviour contexts.

Genetic and environmental interactions over time
Despite size differences at birth, MZ members of multiple sets tend to become more alike with time in physical growth, although the order from tallest to shortest

may not change. Despite early developmental shortfall, the genetic blueprint tends to establish itself in a suitable environment given time.

Psychometric measurements of cognitive development show highly correlated levels of performance for MZ twins, increasing with age. Such data lead to the assumption that 'the genetic blueprint provides back-up capability in the cognitive area when the normal sequence of development has been deflected', or that 'intelligence unfolds in accordance with a genetic timetable for brain development and the timing of particular phases is similar for MZ twins' (Wilson 1977).

In the area of personality development both similarities and differences have been reported. For Smith's (1976) sample of MZ twins, behaviour responses interacted with environmental opportunities in a differential manner so that each new interaction produced further modifications of behavioural characteristics, which in turn resulted in even greater differences on each successive encounter. One twin developed dependency, socialization and casualness. The other developed independence, inquisitiveness, diligence and perseverence.

Henderson (1975) suggested that family influences might work toward diversity or similarity:

> One might well expect, for example, that within a family an innately intelligent child might use superior scanning and storage strategies and selectively use certain aspects of his environment that will further develop his intellectual capacity, while a duller sibling in the same family might be selecting less stimulating environmental features in terms of cognitive development. This relationship would produce a positive within-family GE [genotype-environmental] correlation and thus increase apparent genetic influences on the character being measured. Conversely, on many social and personality traits, especially wide phenotypic differences due to underlying genetic expression may be reduced through family pressure toward greater conformity, thus producing a negative GE correlation.

The phenotypic expressions of genes may, theoretically, widen or diminish in range, or even change ranks, depending on the environmental influences (Schaie 1977). In addition, the purpose of special educational or psychological interventions usually is to reduce the correlation between two factors, not to maintain or increase it (Erlenmeyer-Kimling 1975).

Behavioural genetics has emerged as a field which assumes that there are interactions between genetic and environmental factors (Loehlin 1975). Several large-scale longitudinal studies of twins have had this emphasis (*e.g.* the Louisville study—Wilson 1977; and the La Trobe study—Hay and O'Brien 1981). What is emerging from such efforts to study the interaction of genetic and environmental factors is that the task is complicated. For example, birth-order effects have a parent perception component as well as a biological component (Hay and O'Brien 1984). Methods have become available for the better design of studies in behavioural genetics (Eaves 1972), and for the analysis of genetic and environmental effects across time (Eaves and Eysenck 1976) and across variables (Martin and Eaves 1977). Results from such studies will probably alter the interpretation of past results on genetic effects.

> .. we have in some populations a continuously varying behavioural trait, such as intelligence or impulsivity or visual acuity; we have some plain or fancy theoretical model of the underlying genetic and environmental processes that might be responsible for the variation we observe in this trait; and we either try to see how well the model fits the data, relative to

some other model, or we take the model as given and estimate some parameter, like gene frequency, heritability, or the relation of within- to between-family environmental variance.

In principle, quantitative behavioural genetics could include the fitting of a developmental gene–environment model to the variation of a trait over time in an individual. (Loehlin 1975)

Scarr-Salapatek (1971) pointed out that a developmental perspective can uncover genetic timing mechanisms which might not be noticed in cross-sectional research. Questions in developmental psychology refer to changes over time in the organization of behaviour; the perspective is the life-span. Each individual has a genetically regulated timing of puberty and ageing, and MZ and DZ multiples can be used to study similarity in this biological timing in order to estimate the contribution of heredity. Gedda and Brenci (1975) called this 'chronogenetics'.

Fischbein (1977) conducted a physical growth study which was within that framework. Somatic maturation is strongly regulated by genes and one measure used to estimate somatic maturity has been the age of menarche. MZ twins tend to be more similar than DZ twins for the timing of menarche (Petri 1935, Tisserand-Perrier 1953, Gedda and Brenci 1975). This is an easily obtained measure but it applies to only one sex. Fischbein compared this measure with peak growth velocity in height and weight. If these proved to be satisfactory indicators of somatic maturation they would be available for comparison of boys with girls. Growth velocity studies require a longitudinal research design so that the acceleration that occurs before puberty can be captured. A sample of Swedish children, comprising MZ pairs, same-sex and mixed-sex DZ pairs, and controls, was followed from 10 to 16 years. Height and weight measures, and a rating of secondary sex characteristics were made twice a year by school nurses who also asked the girls for the age at which menarche occurred. All girls were also asked at the age of 17 about their menarcheal age as a check by recall. In summary of this study Fischbein wrote:

Evidence of a rather strong genetic regulation of the occurrence of puberty was obtained in the analysis. The maximal height or weight gain (in cm/year or kg/year) seems to be, at least in girls, less influenced by genetic factors than the age at which it appears.

Questions of genetic influence on psychological variables probably will not be answered by case studies of higher multiples. Such questions may be approached by better techniques of statistical analysis on larger samples of twins which have been carefully allocated to zygosity groups. These should yield findings with higher validity than the early twin studies, according to Plomin and Willerman (1975) and Wilson (1977), especially if the interactionist position of behavioural geneticists proves to be productive of better theory, models and methodologies. Such outcomes will have relevance to the study of higher multiples.

Summary

Research on higher multiple sets must proceed in ways which grapple with the following problems:
- ★ opposing world views or theoretical positions on genetic–environmental contributions to development;
- ★ MZ children may not necessarily be genetically identical, and the prenatal and

birth histories need to be carefully constructed to support an MZ claim;
* environments may lead to (i) an increase in similarities within sets, (ii) an increase in differences within sets, (iii) an increase in differences between sets, or (iv) an increase in differences between MZ and DZ pairs within higher multiple sets;
* variables of unknown genetic transmission, such as intelligence and achievement, are likely to involve large genetic–environmental interactions.

Recommendation: emphasis on within-group differences in similar environments
There are some aspects of the questions of environmental influence to which the study of higher multiples might contribute, despite the relative rarity of such groups. A set of four or more children of the same age, growing up in the same home, whether they are mono- or multizygotic, can provide particular opportunities for studying similar and different responses to the home environment, keeping many factors well under control. It is easier to carry out a research which requires close and frequent observation of interactions when the number of settings is reduced. It is also easier to carry out longitudinal research when the number of families is small. So higher multiples might be used in very detailed studies of environmental effects in genetic–environmental interactions.

There are two major types of environmental influence: natural variables in the context of everyday life, and manipulated variables in a programme of instruction or an experimental treatment. These two aspects of environments are equally important but different in kind. Accepting nature's experiment of higher multiples, the psychologist is in a suitable position to monitor the behavioural consequences on children of particular learning environments or of unusual environmental events or conditions. An example of a 'natural experiment' in school was reported in Chapter 5 (pp. 70–71). The opportunity was created by the splitting of quads into groups of two with two different teachers, acceleration of one group until this became noticeable to the supervising teacher, and then the deliberate acceleration of the other group to bring them up to similar achievement levels. Other examples have been reported by Goshen-Gottstein (1980) in her detailed study of the mothering behaviours of mothers of 'supertwins' (including four sets of quads).

Tunnel (1977) analysed three dimensions of naturalness that can be preserved in research. They are (i) natural behaviour, (ii) natural settings, and (iii) natural treatments. Applying this analysis to research with a multiple set, one could approach the study of:
* natural behaviours, such as language or social play, in naturally occurring settings;
* natural settings, at home, kindergarten or school;
* naturally occurring tasks, problems or learning opportunities;
* natural treatments such as school instruction, or rearing practices in the home.

When a researcher is studying one set of four or more children who are easily followed into different settings, there is the opportunity to test out variations from one environment to another in (i) phenotypic expressions of genetic variables, or (ii) psychological achievements, or (iii) behavioural response patterns. Do the differences between the multiples widen or diminish over time? Does the rank order of the children change on some psychological variable in different settings?

An interesting example of an experimental study was reported by Mountjoy (1957). He conducted a two-day investigation of a pair of MZ twins who, starting from the same magnitude of illusion on the Müller–Lyer task (a linear illusion problem), quickly developed marked divergence from each other *under identical experimental conditions*. He observed that:

★ small differences in reactional biography play an important role in subsequent differential response;

★ the same environment may have quite different functional characteristics for different individuals, even MZ twins;

★ hereditary structures that are nearly identical develop different interactional histories.

He questioned whether such structures play any causal role in behaviour beyond that of being a necessary condition for enabling behaviour to develop. We cannot avoid genetic effects or influences by adopting that position but there would be profit in studies of learning of tasks in the way that Mountjoy worked, or with behaviour analysis methods which provide good research designs with a small sample. In such studies experimental control would need to be established by the design of questions and comparisons in relation to:

★ the zygosity mix of the set and the likelihood of genetic similarity in MZ sets;

★ the possibility that individuals in the set had had different experiences;

★ the medical histories of individuals in the set, particularly where these had been different;

★ the developed abilities of the individuals in the set (general or specific);

★ the contingencies that operate for individuals in a set, particularly where these are different.

Even when the atypical status of a higher multiple set is thought to be a threat to external validity there are some interesting comparisons to be made when there is one atypical member of an otherwise normal set; the normality of the remaining children is thrown into clearer perspective.

APPENDIX 1

QUADRUPLET BIRTHS IN THE LITERATURE: A CATALOGUE OF CASES

*Compiled by Marie M. Clay and Pat Chappelle**

This catalogue comprises all the cases of quadruplet births that we have been able to track down in the literature, up to the first recorded live delivery—in January 1984—of quads conceived by *in vitro* fertilization. No claim is made for its completeness: many medical reports are confined to obscure and hard-to-find journals (about 20 early reports listed in the *Index Medicus* could not be located), and newspaper reports are, of course, even more elusive. Naturally it represents only a fraction of cases. Many births have gone unreported, and news of others will have been withheld due to concern about the effects of publicity. Where cases remained anonymous or where an assumed name had been given, it was often difficult to discern where two or more separate reports were in fact referring to the same set. Entries are arranged in chronological order—where possible, of birth, or else of first report. Pertinent details of birth, zygosity and postnatal histories are given, as well as source references, and photographs have been reproduced where available. With only one exception—the remarkable case of Feodor Vassilyev, related in the plate overleaf—there is no recorded instance of the same mother giving birth to more than one set of quads in her lifetime.

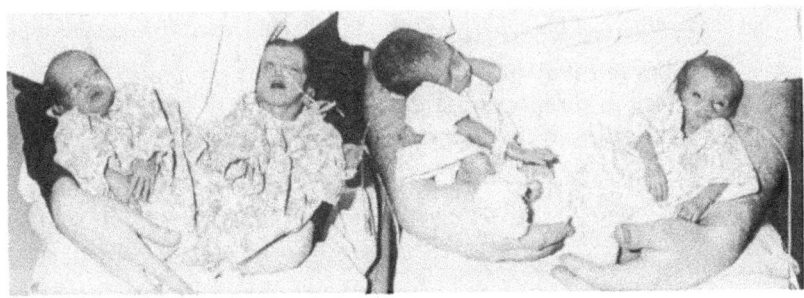

*Special thanks for their help in compiling this Catalogue to: Dorly Barnsley, Hans Everts, Olive Johnson, Hans-Peter Stoffel and Roger Peddie, for assistance with German, Dutch, Spanish, Russian and French translations; Frances Price of the Child Care and Development Group, University of Cambridge; Sheila Goldsmith and Susannah Adams of Guinness Books for allowing us access to the files of the *Guinness Book of Records* (all information used from this source is copyright ©1989 Guinness Publishing Limited); and the ever-patient staff of all the medical libraries employed throughout this research, in particular that of the Royal Society of Medicine, London.

FEODOR VASSILYEV: A CASE OF REMARKABLE FECUNDITY

The case of a Russian peasant, who by 1782 had had, by two wives, a total of 87 children, including four sets of quads, is often cited. In a wide-ranging historical review, Bell (1933) quotes a contemporaneous account published in *The Gentleman's Magazine* (1783, **53**, 753):

"In an original letter now before me, dated St Petersburg, Aug. 13, 1782, O.S., Feodor Wassilief [*sic*], aged 75, a peasant, said to be now alive and in perfect health, in the Government of Moscow, has had—

By his first wife:	By his second wife:
4 × 4 = 16	6 × 2 = 12
7 × 3 = 21	2 × 3 = 6
16 × 2 = 32	8 births 18 children
27 births 69 children	

In all 35 births, 87 children, of which 84 are living and only three buried. . . . The above relation, however astonishing, may be depended upon, as it came directly from an English merchant at St Petersburg to his relatives in England, who added that the peasant was to be introduced to the Empress."

Despite both its seeming improbability, and the various distortions that have appeared in accounts from time to time, most commentators have concurred in the belief that there must be some truth to the story. The definitive reference would appear to be Bashutskiy's (1834) volume *Saint Petersburg Panorama*, which notes that:

In the day of 27 February 1782, the list from Nikolskiy monastery came to Moscow, containing the information that a peasant of the Shuya district, Feodor Vassilyev, married twice, had 87 children. His first wife in 27 confinements gave birth to 16 pairs of twins, seven sets of triplets and four sets of quadruplets. His second wife in eight confinements gave birth to six pairs of twins and two sets of triplets. F. Vassilyev was 75 at that time with 82 of his children alive. [Translation courtesy Guinness Books.]

The case appears in many other sources, notably the *Lancet* (1878), which included the story in a report on a detailed twin study which had 'received honourable mention from the French Academy':

Apropos of this enquiry, the Committee of the Academy recall an account of a quite extraordinary fecundity that was published by M. Hermann in his "Travaux Statistiques de la Russie." Fedor Vassilet [*sic*] . . . who, in 1782, was aged 75 years, had had, by two wives, 87 children.

The family details were repeated as given above, apart from the statement (likely a misprint) that, 'In 1872 [*sic*], 83 of the 87 survived.' The report continued . . .

This fact, almost incredible, is stated to be, nevertheless, authentic. M. Khanikoff, correspondent of the Imperial Academy of St. Petersburg, was consulted, a few years ago, as to the means to pursue in order to obtain a verification of the phenomenon. He replied that all investigation was superfluous, that the family in question still existed in Moscow and that it had been the object of favours from the Government.

Sadly, this evasion of a proper investigation seems, in retrospect, to have dealt a terminal blow to our chances of ever establishing the true detail of this extraordinary case.

Башуцкий, А.П. (1834) Панорама Санкт-Петербурга, Т.2, Спб, 1.
Bell, J. (1933) 'Plural births with a new pedigree.' *Biometrika*, **25**, 110–120.
Lancet (1878) 'Twins.' **1**, 281–290.

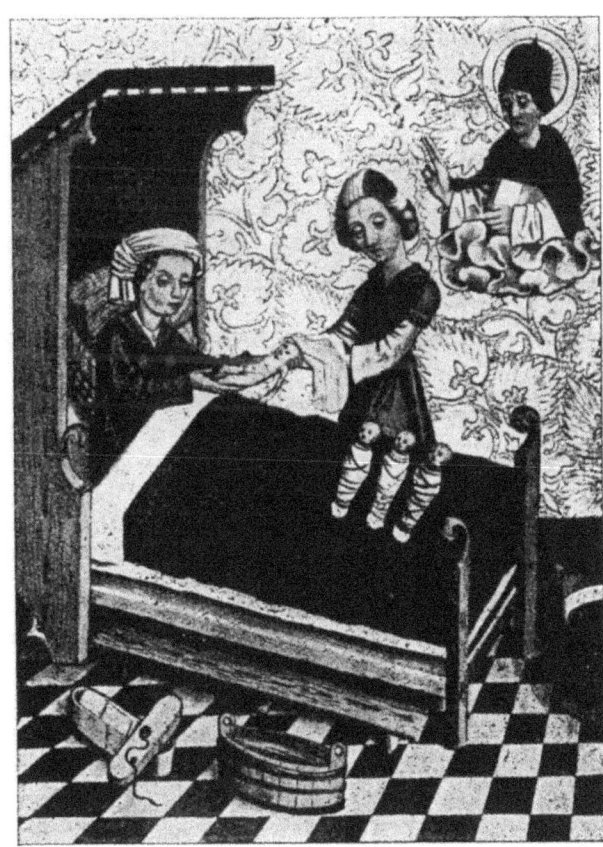

Fifteenth century engraving depicting the delivery of quads. The practice of swaddling was common in Europe up to the beginning of the 19th century

ANON., *?Italy, c.1830—all stillborn.*
Von Winckel (1904) is a secondary source of a case, reported by Panizza (1830, not seen), of a set of non-viable quads, which were preserved in the museum of Pavia, Italy. They were reported to be monochorionic: 'from the same blastoderm must have come two single fruit and a double-monster'.

Panizza (1830) *Präparat des anatomischen Museums zu Pavia.*
von Winckel, F. (1904) *Handbuch der Geburtshülfe*, Band 1, Hälfte II. Wiesbaden: J.F. Bergmann.

ANON., *Germany, May 1847—all surviving birth, one still alive at 24 years.*
Leopold (1871), in connection with a report on quads born in Glauchau in November 1870, mentioned this four-girl set, born in the neighbouring town of Crimmitzschau. The mother had seven previous births, and subsequently one more, all 'easy and happy'. All the quads survived the birth (no details were given except that there was a single placenta), but one died of bronchial pneumonia at 1½ years, another of scarlet fever at 7 years, and a third of typhus at 20 years. The fourth was still alive at the time of Leopold's report.

Leopold (1871) 'Eine Vierlingsgeburt.' *Archiv für Gynaekologie*, **2**, 285–288.

ANON., *Germany, 19 June 1869—none surviving.*
The mother, who lived in the town of Glauchau, was 27 years old and had had four children (all singletons) previously. The family was very poor: she stated that for the last few months of her pregnancy she had lived on nothing but bread and coffee. She gave birth at home—on the floor, as the beds were in hock—with the assistance of a midwife. The quads (two boys and two girls) were delivered in the space of 45 minutes. Their birthweights were around 905, 655, 705 and 750g respectively. It was later reported (Leopold 1871) that they all died shortly after birth.

Leopold (1869) 'Bericht über eine Vierlingsgeburt.' *Monatsschrift für Geburtskunde und Frauenkrankheiten*, **34**, 437–441.
—— (1871) 'Eine Vierlingsgeburt.' *Archiv für Gynaekologie*, **2**, 285–288.

ANON., *Germany, 30 November 1870—none surviving past 21 days.*
This was the second quadruplet birth in the town of Glauchau in consecutive years. The mother was 34 years old and already had five healthy children. These quads—all girls—were born eight weeks preterm; the birthweights ranged from 1300 up to 1433g. Because the mother's milk dried up, a wet-nurse was taken on. At first the infants appeared to be thriving. Their voices became strong, and the wet-nurse claimed she could tell them apart because each had a different sound. However, in the second week they visibly regressed and despite all efforts they died—the first-born at 12 days, the third at 20 days, and the second and fourth at 21 days.

Leopold (1871) 'Eine Vierlingsgeburt.' *Archiv für Gynaekologie*, **2**, 285–288.

ANON., *Germany, 15 April 1878—none surviving.*
The mother was 32 years old and had had five children previously. There was no history of twinning on the mother's side of the family. The quads, two girls and two boys, were born very preterm: the first stillborn, the others surviving no more than a few minutes. The heaviest weighed only 460g. There was one placenta. They were diagnosed to be a TZ set, the two boys being MZ 'twins'.

Müller, P. (1878) 'Eine Vierlingsgeburt.' *Zeitschrift für Geburtshulfe und Gynäkologie*, **3**, 166–172.

GEHRI, *Switzerland, 26 September 1880—all surviving.*
The Gehri quads appear to be the first (authenticated) case on record of a set of quads surviving to adulthood. Their birth was briefly reported by Glaser (1881), who noted that the combined birthweight was 6700g and that, from the appearance of the placenta, they were probably a QZ set. They soon became ill and atrophic, and one suffered sclerema, but all responded well to treatment. A note, published in the *Correspondenz-Blatt für Schweizer Aerzte* after a visit to the quads, noted:

They are now 8 months old, growing much stronger in the fresh air . . . they are bathed frequently and their only food is good cow's milk—not only from consideration of hygiene but also on eminently practical grounds, because they are all able to drink from their bottles, while soup or puree, fed to them by spoon, takes too much time.

The children, two boys and two girls, are healthy and the size of 5-month-olds. Their complexions are somewhat pallid, bone development normal. The last-born is somewhat smaller, thinner and paler than the others, but healthy . . . It is heartwarming to note how the mother tends the children with such care, and how the father regards it as an honour to be the father of quads.

Schlaginhaufen, a Swiss professor with an interest in multiple births, discovered the Gehris during the 1930s, all still in full health. He made an extensive study of their physical characteristics and genealogy, publishing his findings in a comprehensive report in the *Archiv der Julius Klaus-Stiftung* in 1940.

The birth occurred at Oberlindach, in the canton of Bern. The mother (b. Elizabeth von Büren) was 39 years old and already had three children from her previous marriage to Christian König, who died in 1877. She is described as 'a strong countrywoman'. Her husband, Karl Gehri, was a 'painter' (whether this means an artist or house painter is not clear). The first-born, Oskar, was delivered at 6am, but the other three (Bertha, Rosa and Arthur) did not arrive until between 10.30 and 12.30. From a diary kept by the midwife (one Frau Haller, who stayed on with the family, nursing the quads, for seven months after the birth), the individual birthweights were found to be as follows: Oskar, 2080g; Bertha, 1330g; Rosa, 1730g; Arthur, 1580g. The period of gestation was at least 8½ months, and according to the midwife birth occurred in the 38th week. The mother had three further pregnancies, at two-year intervals, each time producing a single baby.

Schlaginhaufen reported in great detail on the physical measurements and differential growth characteristics of the quads, including comparisons with their four surviving siblings. Also featured in the article were several photographs of the quads (at ages 2 to 60 years; see overleaf and p. 14) and of their parents and siblings, plus individual letters from each of the quads, detailing their life history.

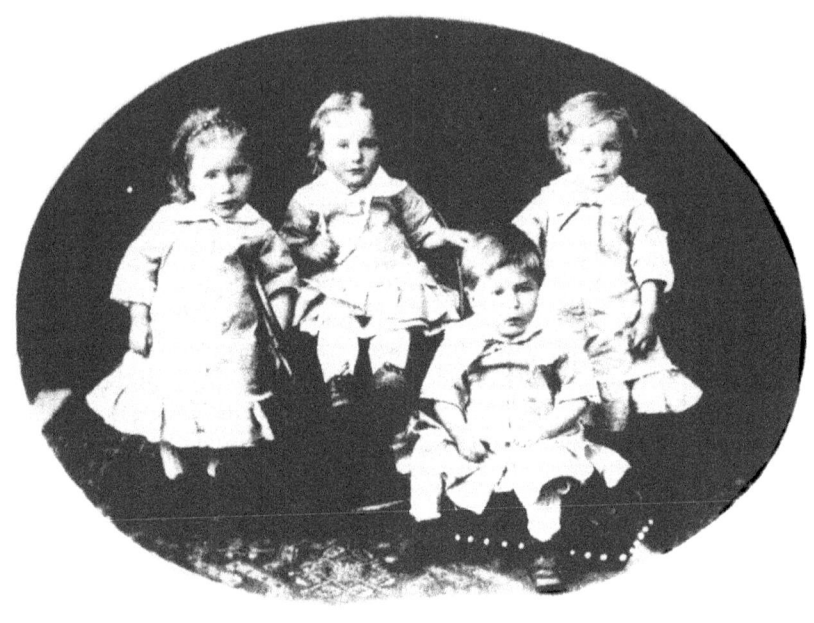

The **Gehri** quads, the first known set to survive to adulthood: *above,* at about 2 years (*l–r,* Rosa, Bertha, Oskar, Arthur); *below,* at 16½ years (*l–r,* Rosa, Oskar, Bertha, Arthur);

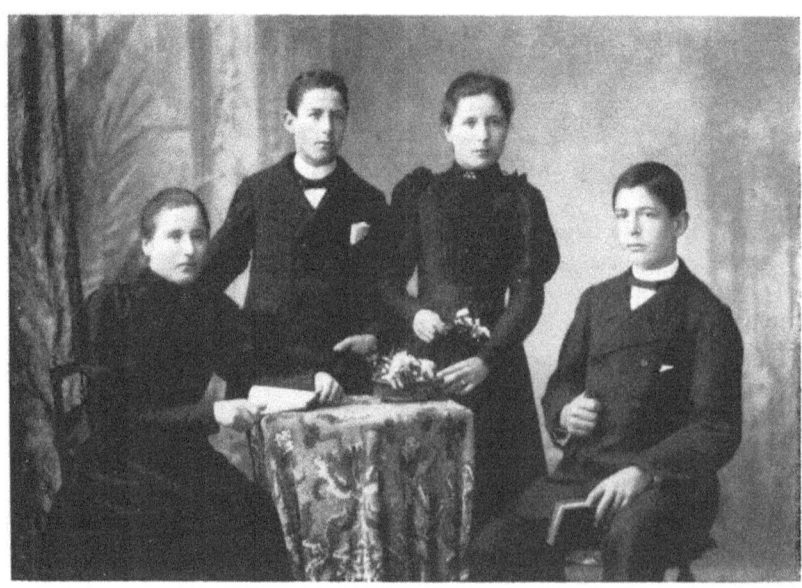

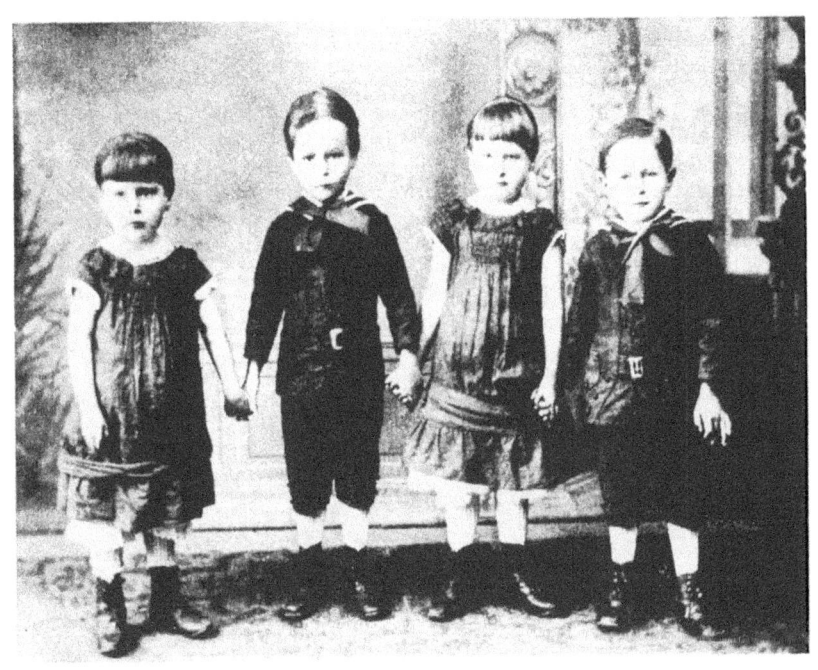

above, age 6 years (*l–r,* Bertha, Arthur, Rosa, Oskar); *below,* age 28 years (*l–r,* Oskar, Rosa, Arthur, Bertha) (all photos from Schlaginhaufen 1940)

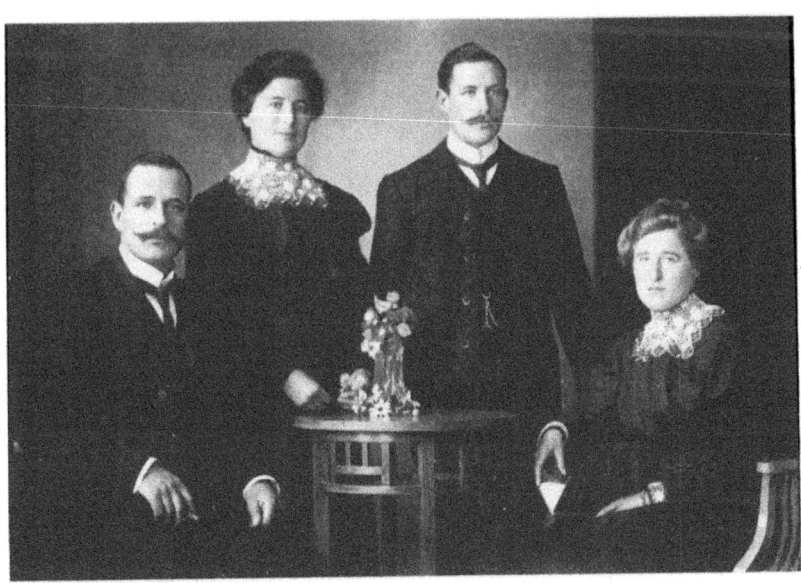

In addition, their genealogy was illustrated with 10 family trees, centring on different branches of the family and revealing a considerable history of twinning. This was summarized in a subsequent report by Spillman (1941):

The mother of the quadruplets has twinning seven times in the paternal collateral lines and five times in the maternal, and she is furthermore the maternal grandmother of two pairs of twins. She is without doubt a homozygotic bearer of the trait. For the father of the quadruplets it could only be shown that he is the son of a mother who was herself a twin, and that only one pair of twins is found in his maternal collateral lines together with the descendents of his siblings. (Spillman 1941)

It was quite remarkable to find a set of quadruplets all alive at 60 years, having survived pregnancy, natal and neonatal hazards in 1880.

Correspondenz-Blatt für Schweizer Aerzte (1881) 'Die Vierlinge.' **11**, 537–538.
Glaser (1881) 'Ein Fall von Vierlingsgeburt.' *Correspondenz-Blatt für Schweizer Aerzte*, **11**, 302.
Schlaginhaufen, O. (1940) 'Die Vierlingsgeschwister Gehri und ihr Verwandtschaftskreis. Eine Familienanthropologische Untersuchung.' *Archiv der Julius Klaus-Stiftung für Vererbungsforschung, Sozialanthropologie und Rassenhygiene*, **15**, 309–398.
Spillman, R. (1941) 'A study of the genetics of twinning, in a family with quadruplets.' *Journal of Heredity*, **32**, 401.

RATTENBURY, *Australia, 19 June 1888—none surviving.*

The mother, who was 31 years old, lived at Tempe, near Sydney, and had had seven children previously, all term singletons. Before this birth she was 'an immense size, in fact a burden to herself near the last, feet and legs very oedematous'. She was taken ill five days before the birth, during which time she felt an occasional pain. Onset of labour was spontaneous, with rupture of the membranes containing the first child, taking the husband by surprise. As he helped her to bed, the baby was expelled. He immediately called the midwife, who arrived within five minutes. She had only just tied the baby's cord when the second child was expelled, followed by a placenta with two cords attached. The third and fourth babies were born within only a few more minutes, each with a single placenta. The children, three girls and a boy, were all born alive, and were 'as large as the usual 5½ month child, perfectly formed and exceedingly well nourished'. They lived from 2 to 6½ hours. The mother's doctor was called the next day because she was suffering from severe after pains and very painful haemorrhoids. She made an uninterrupted recovery, and was out of bed on the 11th day. In a postscript to the report, the editor described the case as 'sufficiently remarkable . . . to strike terror into the hearts of nervous married men as to the possible risks they have undertaken when venturing on matrimony'.

Breneman, P.P. (1888) 'An unusually rare case of plural births.' *Australasian Medical Gazette*, **7**, 273.

DEBIE, *Belgium, 11 August 1888—two born alive.*

The mother had had 10 previous pregnancies and one miscarriage at 3 months; only four of the children were still living. There was no history of plural births on either side of the family. This pregnancy was beset with several complications. The mother grew very rapidly and walking eventually became impossible. She became so unwell that she was confined to bed and given the last rites. It had been decided not to engage a midwife to assist at the birth; however, when labour began unexpectedly at around the eighth month, it was impossible to transport the mother to hospital and two accoucheuses—Mmes Havasse and Wtterwulghe—were urgently summoned by the husband. Mme Havasse was the first to arrive; she found the first child already born, and cradled in the lap of a neighbour, the birth membranes still attached. A boy, it had survived only a few minutes, having asphyxiated because no-one had thought to break open the membranes. The second baby presented shortly after Mme Wtterwulghe arrived. The mother was given some wine and cognac to drink, and the baby, another boy, was extracted. The third and fourth babies were both girls; delivery was much more difficult, demanding manual extraction, and the last one died as it was born. The membranes followed soon after: a single placenta and then a mass comprising two more placentae. In all, the labour had taken three-and-a-half hours. The two surviving infants each weighed about 2kg; a week after the birth they and the mother appeared to be progressing well.

Havasse and Wtterwulghe (1888) 'Grossesse quadruple; oedème considérable; accouchement près du terme de quatre enfants bien développés, deux garçons et deux filles: deux mort-nés, deux vivants. Suites heureuses.' *Journal d'Accouchements*, **9**, 181–183.

ANON., *England, 3 November 1888—none surviving.*
This case occurred in the village of Monkwearmouth, Sunderland. The doctor, summoned to attend a woman in labour, arrived to find her 'on her hands and knees on the floor, with a child just newly born with its cord still unligatured'. Having tied this off and helped the mother into bed, he discovered by digital examination a second amniotic sac whose descent was hindered by the absence of any uterine effort. After he had delivered this child the labour pains returned, though at first only weakly, and the third and fourth children were delivered soon after. All were 'perfectly formed in every respect, even to the nails on the fingers and toes', weighing between 1135 and 1360g. They were in separate amniotic sacs, with one 'extremely large' placenta. From the mother's calculations they were born about a month preterm. As the report concluded, 'The children, it is hardly necessary to add, all died soon afterwards'—the last two, being rather weaker, living for 20 and 21 hours, and the first two for 43 and 44 hours. The sex of the babies was not recorded; the mother's age was given as 'about 35 years'. In a footnote, the doctor added 'I had the honour a few days afterwards to receive from Her Majesty on behalf of the mother a donation of £3.'

Somerville, W. (1888) 'A case of quadruplets.' *British Medical Journal*, **2**, 1386.

ANON., *Germany, 5 November 1888—none surviving.*
For the mother, who was 26 years old, this was her first pregnancy, though by her description of her menstruation prior to this conception, it is possible that she may have had an early miscarriage a short time before. Twins were suspected as early as the fourth month because of her size. The first-born, a girl, lived for only five

minutes, while the other three (two more girls and a boy) were all stillborn. The birthweights were 770, 745, 750 and 800g. There were two placentae, each with two amnions—the first monochorionic, the second dichorionic—and these were described in some detail. There was a history of twinning on both sides of the family.

Steffeck (1888) 'Eine Vierlingsgeburt.' *Centralblatt für Gynäkologie*, **12**, 844–847.

ANON., *Wales, 5 March 1889—none surviving.*
The mother had had three previous confinements, all normal. She first saw her doctor at the beginning of February, complaining of difficulty of breathing. She was very swollen, with emphysematous lungs and a weak heart. By appearance she was approaching full term, though she thought she had another three months to go. She was confined to bed until the birth, during which time her condition continued to deteriorate. The first baby arrived early in the morning of March 5th. There were no previous labour pains, the mother having merely felt an urge to micturate. An hour later the second infant delivered itself, and in another half an hour the remaining two. The last-born, who died soon after birth, was accompanied by the large coalesced placenta of itself and the first two; all three were female, and appeared to have reached full term. The third baby was delivered with its own, separate placenta; it was stillborn, smaller than the others and 'arrested morphologically in its development, having its lower extremities so completely webbed that it was not possible to ascertain the sex.' The mother died about six hours after the last birth, 'from shock, brought on principally through cardiac inadequacy.' The remaining two infants also died, the second-born after 27 hours, the first at 10 days.

Thomas, D. (1889) 'Quadruplets.' *British Medical Journal*, **2**, 194.

NORRISS, *Australia, 28 March 1889—none surviving.*
If the report of this case is accurate, this would be the heaviest recorded set of quads ever born, with a combined birthweight of around 12,700g:

The children, three females and one male, were fully developed, weighing, on average, about 7lbs [3175g] each. . This case is remarkable, as Mrs. N. had previously given birth on one occasion to twins; and also (although recorded in the various works on midwifery, of women having given birth to four and five children at a time, they were generally premature) this woman having, however, in this case, carried the full time, and brought forth perfectly developed offspring.

The babies were all delivered in the space of one hour. The four cords were attached to a single placenta. The mother (who was 34 years old) had considerable pain and diarrhoea after the birth but responded well to treatment and made a full recovery. However . .

The circumstances surrounding the parents, they being poor, precluded their giving the full attention to the children, which was necessary. Two died from atrophy or diarrhoea, within a fortnight, the others within a month, from the same cause; but there can be no doubt had favourable conditions been present there is no reason to suppose other than that this quadruple would have reached maturity.

Robertson, F., Glasgow, L.F.P.S. (1889) 'A case of quadruple birth.' *Australasian Medical Gazette*, **8**, 208–209.

ANON., *2 October 1895—none surviving.*
Where this birth took place is unclear from the medical report: the author was an obstetrician at Rush Medical College, Chicago, but both parents were said to be 'natives' of County Mayo, Ireland. The mother had previously given birth to six children, all singletons, one stillborn, four still living. This birth occurred at home 'under poor circumstances', with a midwife in attendance. According to the mother, gestation was just past the eighth month. The four babies were delivered in about three hours. The placental mass was expelled with the fourth, and comprised four small placentae, united by membranous tissue, each with its own cord and amnio-chorionic sac. The babies—two boys (James, Patrick) and two girls (Bridget, Catharine)—were all living and well-developed, with birthweights of 1135, 1590, 1250 and 1360g respectively. The first three died at 16, 17 and 18 hours postpartum. The photograph, reproduced below, was taken two days later, when the author of the report first saw them. At that stage the

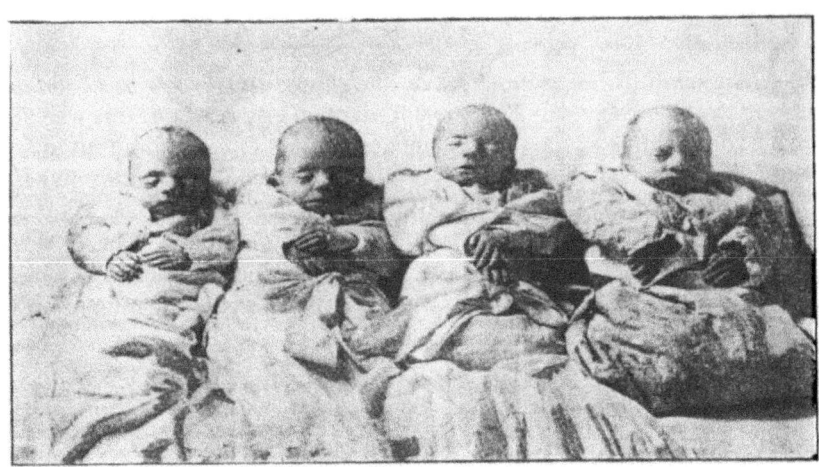

Before the turn of the century few quads survived the neonatal period (Stahl 1895)

fourth infant was moribund, and she subsequently died at 78 hours. In the (somewhat idiosyncratic) report, the mother was said later to be 'about and well with her 180 pounds, actively engaged in selling negatives of her quadruplets. They are very poor.'

Stahl, F.A. (1895) 'A case of quadruplets.' *Journal of the American Medical Association*, **25**, 1038–1040.

ANON., *c.1897—none surviving.*
Saniter (1901, p. 379), in an article concerning MZ triplets, summarized a report by Ausch (1897, not seen) of a set of asymmetrical DZ quads (*i.e.* with three embryos developing from one zygote—see Fig. 1.1, p. 3), born at around six months gestation. Three of the fetuses (all female) were normally developed but the fourth was macerated and decomposing, with a harelip and cleft palate. The mother was 24 years old and had had two previous pregnancies.

Ausch (1897) 'Beitrag zur Casuistik der Vierlingsschwangerschaft.' *Prager Medizinischer Wochenschrift*, **22** (11), 123.
Saniter, R. (1901) 'Drillingsgeburten. Eineiige Drillinge.' *Zeitschrift für Geburtshülfe und Gynäkologie*, **46**, 347–384.

ANON., *England, 22/23 January 1897—all stillborn.*
In this case, the doctor was summoned to the mother's home the day after the birth of the first two babies because 'the "afterbirth" did not come away satisfactorily'. On examination (15 hours after the birth of the 'twins'), a bag of membranes presented which was found to contain a third child; subsequently the fourth was felt and this was born in due course. All the babies were stillborn, at between the fifth and sixth months. There were three distinct placentae and four cords. No details of sex or birthweight were given. It was the mother's third confinement.

Goode, E.T. (1897) 'A case of quadruplets.' *Lancet*, **1**, 590.

ANON., *Netherlands, 27 November 1902—surviving from 4 days to 11 months.*
For the mother, who was aged 25 years and lived in Amsterdam, this was her first pregnancy. The multiple gestation was diagnosed after she was admitted to hospital on 24 November. She was in generally poor health. Labour was induced and lasted two hours. All the babies were girls, and all cried at birth and had good colour. Birthweights were approximately 1200, 1200, 1320 and 1350g. There were four separate placentae and amniotic sacs. All died within their first year, the last at 11 months. The mother recovered slowly—there were some complications and she did not reach full health until the following June.

Van Bergen, J.J.M. (1912) 'Geboorte van een Vierling in de Amsterdamsche Vrouwenkliniek.' *In: Feestbundol opgedragen aan H. Treub* (pp. 395–400).

ANON., *England, 16 September 1904—none surviving.*
The mother was 36 years old and had had five previous pregnancies, all of singletons. She was admitted to the lying-in ward of the St. Pancras Infirmary, London, in the evening of 15 September, having lost a quantity of water after straining to lift a heavy saucepan. She had a good night's sleep feeling 'a few slight niggling pains' at 3am. At 9.30am a child was found to be presenting with one hand prolapsed outside the vagina. The baby, a girl of 565g, was delivered by forceps; she lived for only 13 hours. Within the next 20 minutes three other children,

another girl and two boys, were expelled, all stillborn, the heaviest weighing just 735g. The placentae were delivered after a further 20 minutes. Two were separate, the third being dichorionic with coalescing margins, indicating a QZ origin. By appearance, the babies were of around 6½ months gestational age, though the mother insisted they could be no more than 5½ months. The case was noteworthy for the lack of postpartum haemorrhage, particularly considering the long second stage and the fact that the mother had suffered severely from this complication after two of her previous pregnancies.

Gowdey, A.C. (1904) 'Notes on a case of quadruplets.' *Lancet*, **2**, 1020–1021.

ANON., *Australia, 26 May 1905—three surviving.*
The mother, who lived in Cowra, NSW, was aged 32 years. There was a history of twinning on the maternal side of her family. In six previous confinements she had given birth to twins, triplets (stillborn), a singleton, twins again, and two further singletons, all of whom (aside from the triplets) were still alive at the time of report. In addition, 18 months previously she had had a *placenta praevia* with decomposing fetus removed at five months. Examination by palpation four days before the birth suggested twins 'at least'. The four babies were delivered in just over two hours from the commencement of labour. There were three boys (one stillborn) and a girl, with four separate placentae. The birthweights were not given, but the three surviving infants were said to be 'thriving' at 3 months.

Roberts, L.W. (1905) 'A case of quadruplets.' *British Medical Journal*, **2**, 629–630.

ANON., *USA, 20 December 1906—none surviving.*
The mother lived in Jefferson, MA; she was 31 years of age and this was her first pregnancy. Throughout the pregnancy she was under the direction of the doctor who reported the case (Washburn 1907); his prenatal diagnosis was of twins with hydramnios. Between the fifth and sixth months she gave birth to three girls and a boy in the space of one hour. Each was enclosed in a separate amniotic sac. Pictures of the placentae were published but no birthweights were reported. Two of the babies lived for half an hour, one died soon after delivery and the other was stillborn.

Washburn, F.H. (1907) 'Report of a case of quadruplets.' *American Journal of Obstetrics and Diseases of Women and Children*, **55**, 751–753.

ANON., *USA, 30 May 1907—one surviving at 6 days.*
The mother was a 36-year-old Irish immigrant living in Roanoke, IN. This was her 11th pregnancy; she had previously had two abortions, and three babies had been stillborn. The duration of pregnancy was not stated. Labour was rapid and delivery easy. The first child was a girl, birthweight 1350g; the second was also a girl, 1250g; the third was a boy, 1350g; the fourth was another girl, 1330g. Three died at 2½, 3 and 30 hours respectively, but the fourth was still alive with 'fair prospects' at

6 days. The placenta and amnion structures were described but zygosity status is not clear from these accounts.

Wilking, S.V. (1907a) 'Birth of quadruplets.' *Journal of the American Medical Association*, **49**, 43.
—— (1907b) 'Quadruplets.' *Fort Wayne Medical Journal-Magazine*, **28**, 207.

ANON., Germany, 27 July 1907—all reported as surviving.
This is the second case in the literature involving quads of reportedly enormous size (see also Norriss, 28 March 1889), the recorded birthweights being 5¾ Pfunde (2875g), 6 Pfd. (3000g), 6¼ Pfd. (3125g) and 5½ Pfd. (2750g)—a total of 11,750g. In addition, the placenta was said to weigh 4½ Pfd. (2250g). The mother, who was aged 43 years and had had 11 children previously (of whom 10 were still living), was said to be 'large and of strong build, but not abnormally so'. There was no history of multiple birth on either side of the family. At two months the infants (all male) were said to be 'all well-nourished, fully developed and up to this time thriving very well.' This may be the first report of a surviving set in this century.

Lachmann (1907) 'Vierlingsgeburt.' *Deutsche Medizinische Wochenschrift*, **33**, 1462.

ANON., USA, 19 July 1908—none surviving past 4 days.
The mother lived in Argentine, KS.; she was aged 35 and had had seven children previously, four of whom were still living. When the first baby—a boy—was born, the doctor was surprised to find that the birth cord was in fact four separate cords braided together. The second boy was born in 15 minutes, a girl 30 minutes later and another boy 30 minutes after that. They were all in a macerated condition. Approximate birthweights were 2040, 1590, 1130 and 910g. The first three babies breathed naturally, the fourth having to be assisted. There were two placentae, one with three cords and the other with one. In order of birth, the infants died at 24 hours, 4 days, 8 hours and 18 hours respectively.

Nave, H.A. (1908) 'Birth of quadruplets.' *Journal of the American Medical Association*, **51**, 1869.

ANON., USA, 6 July 1909—none surviving.
The babies were born at 7 months gestational age, at Weston, WV. Two had already been born dead when the doctor arrived; the third and fourth were delivered soon after, each weighing about 1360g—they lived a few hours only. There were four placentae, each with its own cord, joined together by membrane adhesions.

Snyder, G. (1909) 'An odd confinement.' *Eclectic Medical Journal*, **69**, 469.

ANON., England, 5 October 1909—none surviving.
The mother was an outpatient at Queen Charlotte's Hospital, London. She was aged 28, and had already had seven children and three miscarriages. Because she had not menstruated at all while feeding her previous child, she was unsure when

conception had occurred; however, she thought that she was 26 weeks pregnant. She felt movement eight weeks before the onset of labour. The first two babies, both male, were born dead. The third was a girl who lived 5½ hours and the last child was another boy who lived only 30 minutes. The birthweights were approximately 300, 310, 510 and 510g respectively. From the placental evidence it was judged that this was a TZ set, the first two boys being MZ 'twins'.

White, C. (1910) 'Quadruplets born at the twenty-sixth week.' *Proceedings of the Royal Society of Medicine*, **3** (Obstetrical and Gynaecological Section), 79.

ANON., *30 April 1910—early miscarriage.*
The mother had had 10 children and one miscarriage previously (all single pregnancies). She lost these babies at three months. Three were quite well developed. The fourth embryo was shrivelled and headless and seemed to have been dead for some time. There were marked differences in the sizes of the fetuses.

Willett, J.A. (1910) 'Placenta and membranes of quadruplets.' *Proceedings of the Royal Society of Medicine*, **3** (Obstetrical and Gynaecological Section), 80.

ANON., *Germany, 15 November 1911—none surviving.*
The mother was a 29-year-old peasant of Rostock, Germany. This was her fifth pregnancy following four spontaneous births. She 'grew like a house' from the 12th week onwards, and before the birth was almost incapable of working in the fields as she was so out of breath and sore. The midwife expected a multiple birth; labour began at around 28 to 30 weeks and the babies arrived very rapidly. The first two were boys, weighing 1500 and 1000g; the latter pair were girls, weighing 1000 and 1040g. All died within 25 hours. The doctor, who visited the mother the next day, described her as a strong woman in good health. He considered the children to have been too small and weak to have survived even in a clinic with incubators and skilled personnel. He checked the weights and heights and photographed the dead babies. After carefully questioning the midwife he concluded that they were a TZ set, the girls being MZ 'twins' sharing a single chorion and a single amnion.

Hauser, H. (1913) 'Vierlinge und Vierlingsmütter.' *Muenchener Medizinische Wochenschrift*, **60**, 812–815.

ANON., *USA, 5 August 1912—all surviving at 4 months.*
The midwife attending this birth in Boston, MA, reported:

.. into this unfriendly world, but into the hands of kindly people came one tiny baby, then a second little stranger, then to the astonishment of the doctor and nurses came a third and after a short delay, came the fourth, the largest and prettiest of the sisters.

The four-girl set was born at around 7½ months gestation. Birthweights ranged from 1360 to nearly 1810g, with an aggregate weight of 6350g. There was only one placenta: no further details are provided. The parents had one other child, a son of 5 years. The father was informed after the birth that there were four infants but the mother was told that she had twins—it was not until the day before she went home that she knew she had quads. The babies were fed using expressed milk from the mother supplemented by supplies from wet nurses, and were making good progress at 4 months. One gains the impression that they were still in the local hospital at that time, and that the mother came to feed two every day.

Boswall, E.O. (1912) 'The nursing of quadruplets.' *American Journal of Nursing*, **13**, 342–344.

ANON., *Germany, 9 August 1912—aborted at five months.*
The mother, who was 37 years old, had previously had 'nine births always with only one fruit and two miscarriages in addition'. She was admitted to hospital on August 6th, around the fifth month of pregnancy, with acute hydramnios. She was also severely cyanotic, and two days later it was decided to induce labour by injection of pituitrin. Her waters broke at midnight, and 90 minutes later a fetus of 20cm length was ejected. Three larger fetuses were expelled after a further four hours. The quads were all female and there was a single placenta. MZ diagnosis was supported by macro- and microscopic examination.

Lindig, P. (1913) 'Berichte aus Gynäkologischen Gesellschaften. 1. Freie Vereinigung mitteldeutscher Gynäkologen. (No. 7).' *Zentralblatt für Gynäkologie*, **37**, 70–71.

ANON., *Australia, 14 December 1912—none surviving.*
The mother, who lived in Gilgandra, NSW, was 31 years of age and this was her fourth confinement. She was very large for dates and labour began two months before the expected time. Her previous labours had been severe and abnormal. She was admitted to hospital in labour. After 17 hours the first child, a boy, was delivered by forceps. Chloroform had been given. This procedure was repeated six hours later for a second boy, and after a further 13 hours for the third child, a girl. Shortly after that the fourth child, a stillborn girl, was extracted by forceps. Two placentae were removed manually: the first was very large and had three cords and three bags of membranes attached to it; the second was small and belonged to the stillborn girl. All four infants were of equal size, and at a developmental stage which was in agreement with the mother's dates. Each weighed about 1810g. The first three babies lived for 5, 38 and 65 hours respectively.

Peet, H. (1913) 'A case of multiple pregnancy, quadruplets.' *Australasian Medical Gazette*, **33**, 620.

ANON., *Sweden, 11 March 1913—two surviving.*
The 32-year-old mother lived in Trelleborg in southern Sweden. She was herself a twin, and her grandmother and a sister had also given birth to twins. She already had four children (all singletons—three girls and a boy). She was admitted to hospital two days before the birth. The four babies—all boys—were delivered in the space of 45 minutes, the mother being conscious throughout. Birthweights were 2400, 3270, 1980 and 2720g respectively, the third baby being stillborn. The first

subsequently failed to thrive and died at 5 weeks, but the remaining pair gained weight rapidly. A photograph of all four babies, taken on the second day after the birth, accompanied the report. They were apparently a QZ set. There were two placentae, one with three separate amniotic sacs.

Brattström (1914) included in his report on this set a table listing details of all known quadruplet births in Sweden from 1867 onwards; this table (in adapted form) is reproduced overleaf.

Brattström, E. (1914) 'Ein Fall von viereiigen Vierlingen nebst einigen Beobachtungen betreffs der Vierlingsgeburten im allgemeinen,' *Monatsschrift für Geburtshilfe und Gynäkologie*, **40**, 53–69.

ANON., *France, 7 January 1915—one surviving to 16 years, three still alive at 33.*
This case of quads born in Vendée, France, was reported to the Medical Academy of France in 1920 when the quads were 5 years old. The mother already had six children, four boys and two girls. The midwife examined her one month before the birth and diagnosed a multiple pregnancy. She spent the last month of the pregnancy in bed. The membranes broke spontaneously but the labour contractions were weak and the doctor was called. He delivered the first baby by forceps; this was a girl weighing 1900g. At that time the midwife believed there were two more babies to be born. The second baby, a boy, was delivered by forceps 30 minutes later and weighed 2000g. After a further 30 minutes a vigorous girl, weighing 2050g, was delivered, again by forceps. The fourth baby was a boy born spontaneously and weighing 2100g. The placenta had four distinct pockets.

Progress of the infants was recorded at 2 months and at 4 and 5 years, when they were described as being in good health with 'exceptional parents from all points of view'. The midwife's account, approved by the attending doctor, was reported by Pinard (1920). A further reference to these quads was made by Vaudescal *et al.* (1948). At that time three of the quads were still living aged 33 years, the fourth having been killed in an accident at the age of 16.

Pinard, M. (1920) 'Gestation et accouchement quadruples: enfants viables.' *Bulletin de l'Académie de Médecine de Paris*, **83**, 169–173.
Vaudescal, M.M., Blechmann, G., Levesque, A. (1948) 'Grossesse quadrigémellaire.' *Gynécologie et Obstétrique*, **47**, 883–887.

KEYS, *USA, 4 June 1915—all surviving to adulthood.*
The Keys quads, an all-girl set, were born in Hollis, OK. The mother was 33 years old and had four other children. She breast-fed all four quads until they were 9 months old. At the time of the first report it was thought that they were a DZ set of triplets plus singleton. The second report, entitled 'Women's eyes and potato skins', presented an argument that, despite the fact that three of the girls had blue eyes and the other had brown eyes, they could nonetheless still be an MZ set (the theory being that the characteristic had been inherited by all, but had been 'lost' by one, a phenomenon which had been demonstrated in asexually propagated, purple-skinned potatoes).

QUADRUPLET BIRTHS IN SWEDEN, 1867–1913*

Date of birth	Place of birth	Age of mother	Previous pregnancies	Liveborn ♀	Liveborn ♂	Stillborn ♀	Stillborn ♂	Postnatal status of liveborn children
4 July 1867	Gävleborgs	34	1	2	—	2	—	One died the next day, the other at 3 days
23 March 1871	Kristianstad	43	6	4	—	—	—	All died within 10 hours
4 Oct 1871	Norrbotten	31	—	—	3	—	1	All died within 2 days
10 Jan 1874	Göteborg	24	1	2	1	—	1	One died the next day, the others the day after
1 April 1875	Jämtlands	38	4	1	3	—	—	Three died the same day, the other at 3 days
17 April 1877	Södermanlands	27	2	3	—	—	—	All died within the hour
7 Feb 1878	Stockholm	42	—	—	—	—	2	
12 Sept 1879	Stockholm	25	2	3	—	1	—	Died at 8 days, 12 days, and 3 months
6 Oct 1882	Älfsborg	35	1	1	1	1	1	Both died within the hour
23 Feb 1884	Blekinge	29	5	3	—	1	—	Two died at 10 days, the other at 11 days
5 Dec 1884	Älfsborg	36	2	4	—	—	—	Three died the same day, the other at 3 days
5 Nov 1887	Västmanlands	35	7	2	2	—	—	All died within the hour
20 Oct 1891	Kopparbergs	35	—	1	2	1	—	Not known
22 Dec 1901	Västerbottens	30	4	2	2	—	—	Three died the same day, the other the following day
27 May 1902	Älfsborg	37	4	1	2	—	1	Died at 8 days, 14 days, and 17 days
1 April 1902	Värmlands	34	4	1	3	—	—	The boys died at 3 days, 10 months, and 11 months; the girl survived
19 Jan 1905	Västernorrlands	33	3	3	—	—	1	All died within the day
22 May 1905	Kalmar	36	—	2	—	2	—	Not known
11 March 1913	Malmöhus	32	4	—	3	—	1	See Catalogue entry, pp. 110–111

*Adapted from Brattström (1914).

When the sisters (Roberta, Mona, Mary and Leota) were 12 years old a comprehensive case study was completed by Brintle (see Chapter 5, pp. 67, 73–74), and physical measurements were reported by Spier (see Table 5.II, p. 48). In 1940 Gardner and Newman determined that the quads were in fact a TZ set. Dermatoglyphic studies compared finger patterns, palm patterns and ridge counts. At that time the Keys were the best-known set of quads in the USA. Gardner and

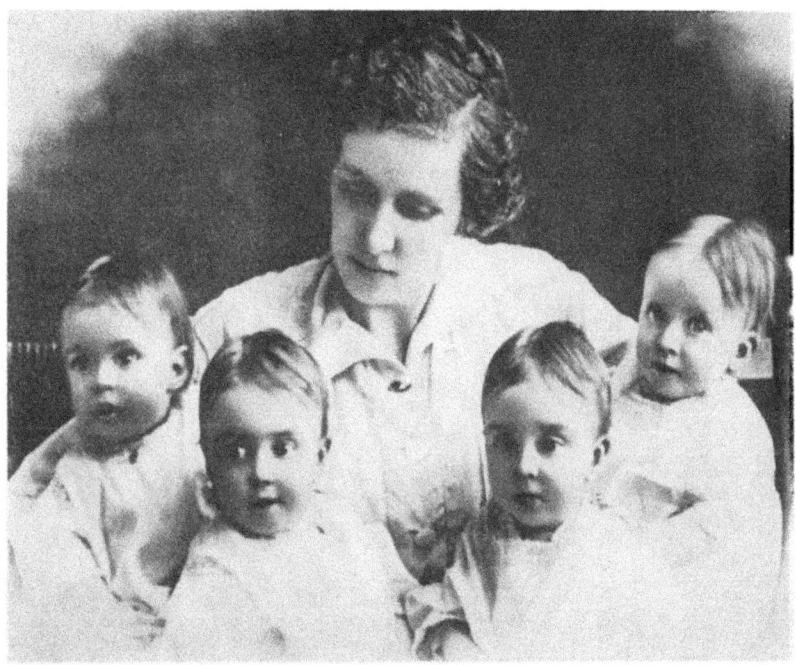

The **Keys** quads, age 1 year (*l–r*, Roberta, Mona, Mary, Leota) (*J. Hered.*, 1916)

Newman later dubbed them the 'College Quadruplets', as 'it seems certain that they are the only *living* set, perhaps the *only* set of quadruplets, who have ever graduated as a complete group from college' (Baylor University in Waco, TX). They appeared in public on many occasions as goodwill ambassadors of the Oklahoma legislature (see Chapter 1, p. 4). Personality tests were interpreted to mean that they were normal, well-adjusted girls, despite their quadruplet status and the excessive publicity they had received as a consequence.

Brintle, S.L. (1931) 'Measurements of quadruplets.' *Journal of Genetic Psychology*, **39**, 91–112.
Gardner, I.C., Newman, H.H. (1940) 'Physical and mental traits of the College Quadruplets.' *Journal of Heredity*, **31**, 419–424.
Journal of Heredity (1916) 'Women's eyes and potato skins.' **7**, 475–477.
Spier, L. (1928) 'Measurements of quadruplet girls.' *American Journal of Physical Anthropology*, **12**, 269–272.
See also *Psychological Abstracts* (1931, **5**, 3409).

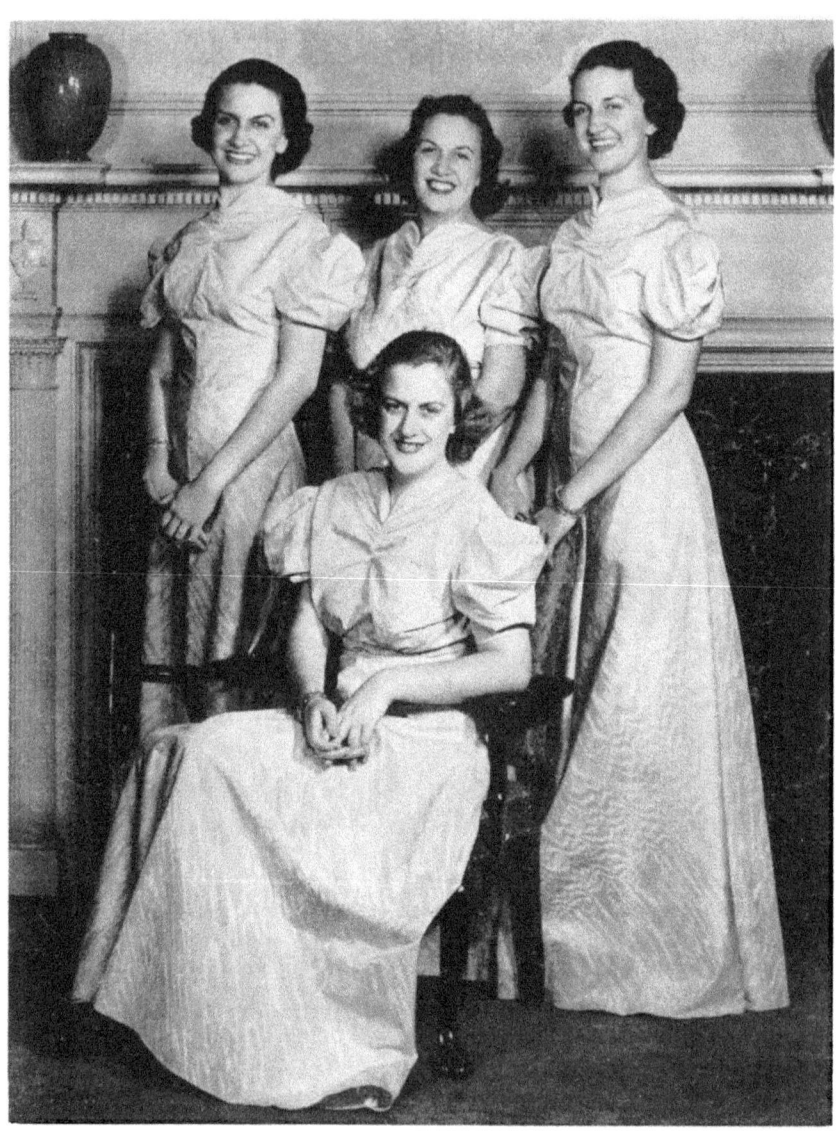

The **Keys** quads (*l–r*, Mona, Mary, Roberta; *seated*, Leota), after having graduated from college (Gardner and Newman 1940)

HALL, *New Zealand, 2 July 1919—two surviving.*
The mother, who was aged 39 years, lived in Ngaruawahia, in the North Island of New Zealand. Dr Harry Caldwell Tait was called to the family home and delivered four preterm babies, all boys. Two died at 8 days. No information is available on the surviving boys. This case history, received in a personal communication from Dr Caldwell Tait's family, was confirmed in a letter from the Registrar General's Office, Lower Hutt, New Zealand.

ANON., *Scotland, 1919—all surviving at time of report.*
A 28-year-old mother in Hamilton, Scotland, gave birth to three boys and a girl at full term. She had had two previous pregnancies of singletons, aged 3 years and nearly 2 years at the time of this birth. There was no history of multiparity on either side of the family. The heaviest of the babies weighed about 2495g and all three others weighed around 2270g. The intervals between the births were 30 minutes, two hours and 10 minutes. There were two placentae, one with three cords and the other with a single cord. The mother and infants were reported to be doing well.

Loudon, J.L. (1919) 'A case of quadruplets.' *British Medical Journal*, **2**, 813.

ANON., *England, reported 1920—none surviving.*
A doctor's son reported the following case which occurred in his late father's practice in Birmingham.

The mother was a primipara, aged 18, and single, and within about two hours gave birth to quadruplets at full time or nearly so. Two were born alive, but died within the day, and of the two born dead one was a monster (preserved in Queen's College, Birmingham). Subsequently the couple married and three or four normal pregnancies ensued, but no further plural birth.

Vinrace, D. (1920) 'Survival of quadruplets.' *Lancet*, **1**, 178. (*Letter*.)

ANON., *USA, 7 November 1923—last surviving to 8 months.*
For the 38-year-old mother, who lived in Baltimore, MD, this was her ninth pregnancy. Labour, which was easy, began several weeks before the calculated date. The first two children, a girl and a boy, were born spontaneously. After medication, the third and fourth children were born, both girls. Birthweights ranged from 2041 to 2269g. All lived for some weeks but the last died at 8 months. The placentae had two chorionic sacs, one belonging to the last born girl, the other a large triple one. As two girls and a boy were attached to this large placenta it must have developed from more than one zygote. Dissection of the membranes showed that each partition wall consisted of four layers—amnion-chorion-chorion-amnion—demonstrating that the quads were quadrizygotic. The report carried a clear and full discussion of the birth membrane analysis, as it was understood at that time (more recent knowledge has refined and corrected this view):

It is now universally admitted that single ovum, or identical, twins are always enclosed within a single chorion, but that an individual amnion surrounds each twin. In other words, the partition wall separating them consists of two layers of amnion, and in rare instances in which it is lacking, it is assumed that it had originally existed and had later become destroyed.
   At present in all well regulated obstetrical services, whenever one has to deal with twins of the same sex attached to a single placenta, the attempt is made to determine whether they are of the single or double ovum variety, by ascertaining whether the partition walls consist of two or four membranes. If the former, both membranes are amnion, whereas in the latter event we have to deal with two amnions and two chorions.

Williams, J.W. (1926) 'Note on placentation in quadruplet and triplet pregnancy.' *Bulletin of the Johns Hopkins Hospital*, **39**, 271–280.

ANON., *France, c.1924—two non-viable; incomplete data on other two.*
The report describes a non-viable MZ pair ('deux jumeaux momifiés dans une même poche amniotique'), plus a DZ pair ('deux jumeaux bivettelins'), the status of whom is not clear. No further details are given.

Lantuéjoul and Reglade (1924) 'Un cas de grossesse quadruple.' *Bulletin de la Société d'Obstétrique et de Gynécologie de Paris*, **13**, 169–170.

DERNER, *Germany, 19 December 1927—all surviving at 8 years.*
The Derner quads, an all-girl set, were born in Beuthen, Germany. There were brief reports in the *Journal of Heredity* on two occasions. Neither of these two reports mentions the mother at all. The first stated that, as the girls were of very similar appearance, 'one suspects that a detailed study of resemblances and differences would demonstrate their origin from a single cell'. However, in the later study, Sarkar reported blood analysis data showing that Quads 1 and 2 were of O, MN blood type, while Quads 3 and 4 were of O, M type, suggesting that they were in fact a symmetrical DZ set (see Fig. 1.1, p. 3). This is the earliest report of the use of blood analysis for zygosity determination that I found in the literature.

Journal of Heredity (1935) 'The Derner quadruplets.' **26**, 256.
Sarkar, S.S. (1943) 'A quadruplet set consisting of two pairs of identical twins.' *Journal of Heredity*, **34**, 283.

ANON., *USA, 7 July 1928—only one live birth.*
The mother was aged 28 years and this was her third pregnancy. She entered hospital (in Rhode Island) a week before the birth. The membranes ruptured spontaneously but labour did not begin for a further four days. The first baby, a boy weighing approximately 2040g, was delivered by forceps. A second boy arrived after the placental mass but was stillborn. The placental tissue consisted of two mature placentae with remnants of their respective membranes, and between them a third, degenerated placenta to which were attached two papyraceous fetuses (see footnote, p. 19). The preterm but viable DZ twins had co-existed with an MZ set of twins whose development had ceased at between three and three-and-a-half months. Such a phenomenon has not appeared in the literature since that time, so this remains an unusual case.

Tartakoff, J. (1930) 'Papyraceous twins in quadruple pregnancy.' *New England Journal of Medicine*, **202**, 78.

ANON., *France, 24 March 1929—all surviving.*
The mother was 33 years old and this was her seventh pregnancy. She had five sons, all living, and a daughter who had died. The gestation proceeded normally until the ninth month. When labour began the midwife thought it was a twin pregnancy. A boy weighing 2300g was delivered first. Then for 20 hours nothing

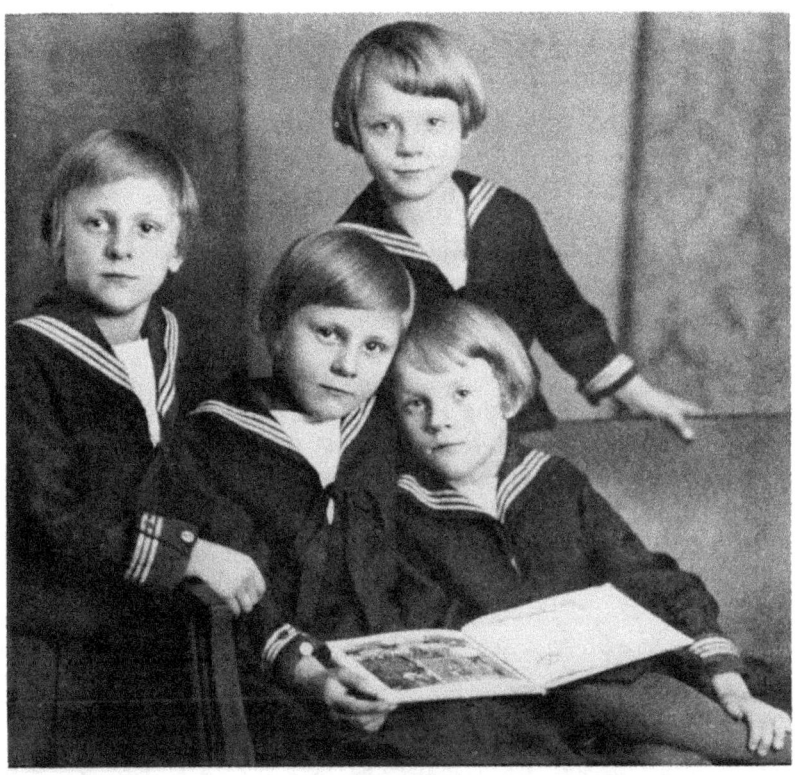

The **Derner** quads (*l–r*, Annelies, Maria, Victoria, Etheltraut) (*J. Hered.*, 1935)

happened and the midwife sent the mother to hospital. A triplet pregnancy was then diagnosed. The next baby was a boy weighing 1750g. Next came another boy, birthweight 2400g, which the doctor believed to be the last baby, until the fourth infant, weighing 1800g (sex not stated), was born. There were four amniotic sacs in pairs inside two chorionic sacs. The mother and children left hospital on the 15th day in excellent condition, the infants having regained their birthweights. The author stated his reasons for reporting the case as: (i) because the gestation was near to full term; and (ii) because the infants survived and were well developed.

Papatestas, N. (1929) 'Gestation quadrigémellaire.' *Bulletin de la Société d'Obstétrique et de Gynécologie de Paris*, **18**, 405–406.

ANON., *Spain, 20 May 1929—none surviving.*
The mother, who already had five children, entered hospital in her seventh month of pregnancy. After the first two boys had been born, a little pressure was applied to remove the placenta. At that time a third boy presented itself, to the surprise of

everyone in attendance. Birthweights for these three babies were 790, 870 and 570g respectively. They lived for only about three hours. Detailed examination of the placenta showed the existence of a *fetus papyraceus* (see footnote, p. 19).

Audebert, J.L., Estienny, E. (1930) 'Grossesse quadrigémellaire.' *Bulletin de la Société d'Obstétrique et de Gynécologie*, **19**, 693–694.

PERRICONE, *USA, 31 October 1929—all surviving at 10 years.*
These quads were highly unusual as an all-male QZ set. The parents were Italian immigrants living on a small farm on the outskirts of Beaumont, TX. There were five older brothers, and one sister who had died. Their weights at birth ranged from 1135 to 1590g. The quads were named Anthony, Bernard, Carl and Donald, giving rise to the collective moniker 'the alphabetical quads'.

Gardner and Newman (1940) reported that there was not much conversation between the father, who did not speak English very well, and the quads, who had not learned Italian—the mother acting as interpreter between them. Despite the parents' efforts to keep the four as similar as possible, they were as unlike each other in every way as were the five older brothers—in fact, 'according to the

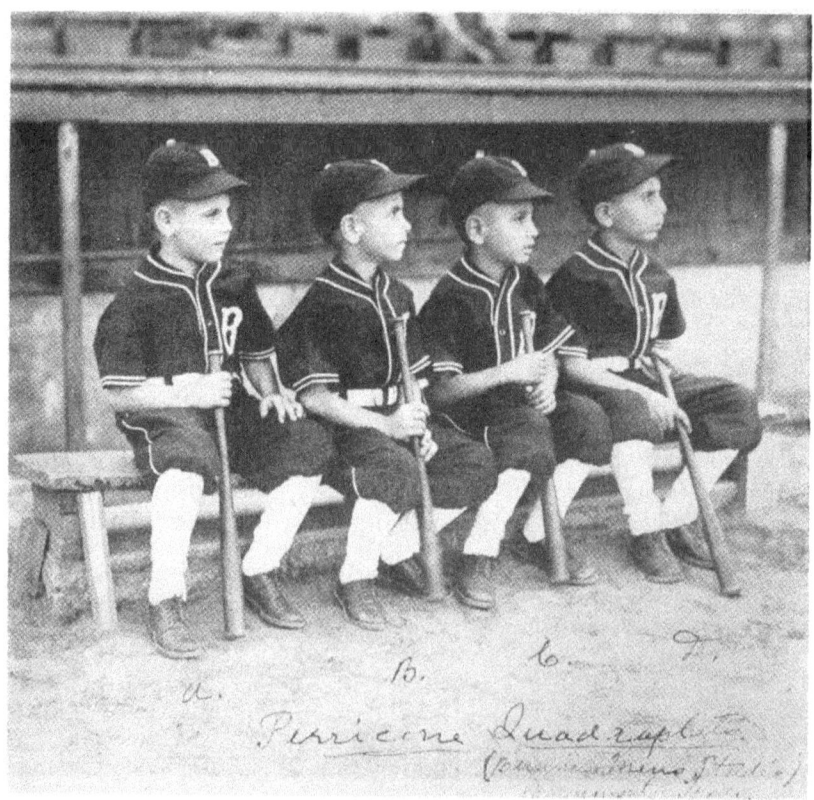

The **Perricone** quads (*l–r*, Anthony, Bernard, Carl, Donald) (Pryor 1936)

mother, who ought to know, each of the quads is more like one of his older brothers than like any other member of his set.'

An extensive study was made of these boys when they were aged about 10 years. Zygosity determination, dermatoglyphic studies, life experiences and mental development were reported by Gardner and Newman, and bone ossification was investigated by Pryor (see Chapter 5, p. 51).

Gardner, I.C., Newman, H.H. (1940) 'The alphabetical Perricone quadruplets: a four-egg set, all males.' *Journal of Heredity*, **31**, 307–314.
Pryor, J.W. (1936) 'Ossification as additional evidence in differentiating identicals and fraternals in multiple births.' *American Journal of Anatomy*, **59**, 409–423.
—— (1939) 'Normal variations in the ossification of bones due to genetic factors.' *Journal of Heredity*, **30**, 249–255.

MORLOK, *USA, 19 May 1930—all surviving.*

The mother was German-Irish, 31 years of age, and lived in Lansing, MI. These quads, all girls, were her only children. The first scientific report came from the Department of Genetics, University of Wisconsin, and did not provide the usual medical history of the pregnancy and birth. According to the attending physician there was only one chorion and they were therefore monozygotic; however, the afterbirth was not preserved for detailed analysis. The birthweights ranged from 1360 to 2040g. A local newspaper ran a competition to find names for the babies. A note, reported by Pryor (1936), from the X-ray technician at the hospital where they were born, explained the winning formula:

The girls' names . . . are Edna A., Wilma B., Sarah C., and Helen D. The first initials of their names are taken from the initials of Edward W. Sparrow Hospital, and their ages are denoted by the initials A, B, C and D.

The family circumstances have been detailed in Chapter 4 (p. 37). When they were 8 months old Clarke (1932) checked them for similarity on genetic markers such as hair colour and kind, eye colour, ear form, palm and sole prints—he thought that the close similarity made it probable that they were an MZ set. Bone ossification studies by Pryor concurred with this diagnosis, as did subsequent tests conducted by MacArthur and MacArthur (1937), Gardner and Newman (1943) and Allen (1960*a*,*b*).

Gardner studied the quads' mental ability, school achievement, and social and personality development at 10 years: the results were interpreted by Newman (who was not a psychologist) as better than satisfactory, and more favourable than the ratings of the Dionne quins who were five years younger. There was a four-month difference in mental age, their rank order for this paralleling that for height and weight. The largest and brightest was seen as the leader (see Chapter 5, p. 72). All were well-adjusted to their community. Their physical characteristics at this age are detailed in Table 5.III (p. 50). At the time of the Gardner and Newman report they were the only surviving MZ quads on record.

Allen, G. (1960*a*) 'The Morlok quadruplets. 1) Probability of uniovular origin judged from qualitative traits.' *Acta Geneticae Medicae et Gemellologiae*, **9**, 240–255.
—— (1960*b*) 'The Morlok quadruplets. 2) The interpretation of quantitative differences.' *Acta Geneticae Medicae et Gemellologiae*, **9**, 452–465.

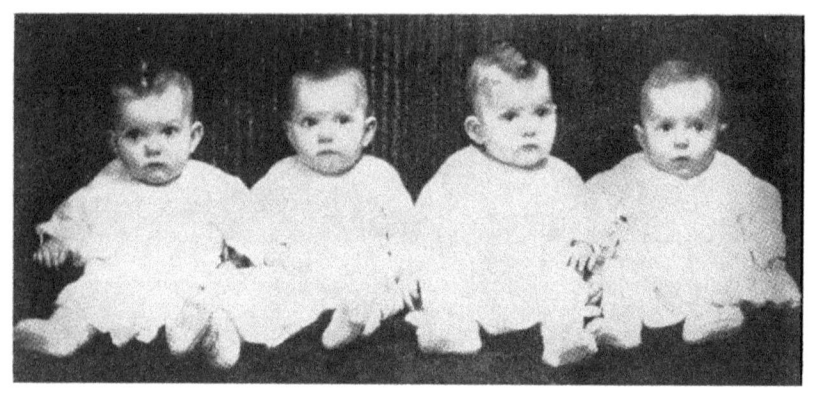

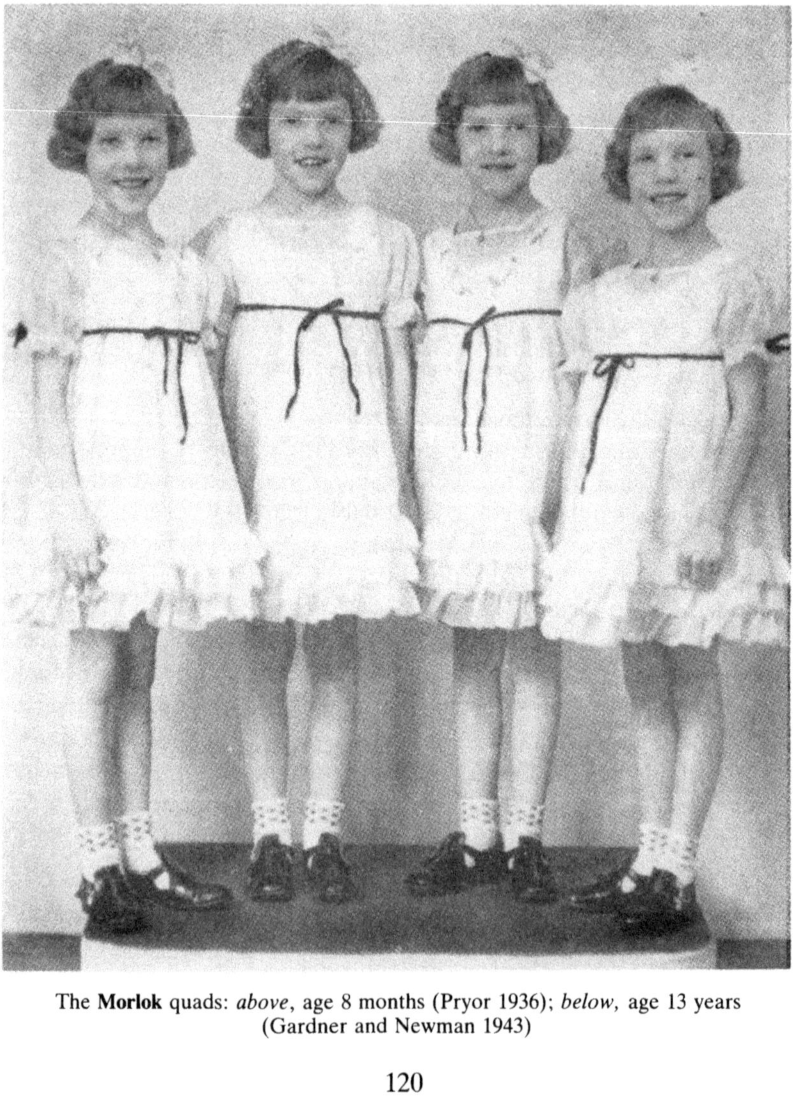

The **Morlok** quads: *above,* age 8 months (Pryor 1936); *below,* age 13 years (Gardner and Newman 1943)

Clarke, A.E. (1932) 'Identical quadruplets.' *Journal of Heredity*, **23**, 257–259.
Gardner, I.C., Newman, H.H. (1943) 'Studies of quadruplets. V—The only living one-egg quadruplets.' *Journal of Heredity*, **34**, 259–263.
Gedda, L. (1951) *Studio dei Gemelli*. Rome: Edizioni Orizzonte Medico.
MacArthur, J.W., MacArthur, O.T. (1937) 'Finger, palm and sole prints of monozygotic quadruplets.' *Journal of Heredity*, **28**, 147–153.
Pryor, J.W. (1936) 'Ossification as additional evidence in differentiating identicals and fraternals in multiple births.' *American Journal of Anatomy*, **59**, 409–423.
—— (1939) 'Normal variations in the ossification of bones due to genetic factors.' *Journal of Heredity*, **30**, 249–255.

SCHENSE, *USA, 13 January 1931—all surviving.*
These quads were born in Aberdeen, SD, about five weeks preterm. From communication with the attending doctor, Pryor (1939) reported that the mother was in labour for four hours 40 minutes, and there were two normal vertex presentations and two assisted births. The condition of the babies was good

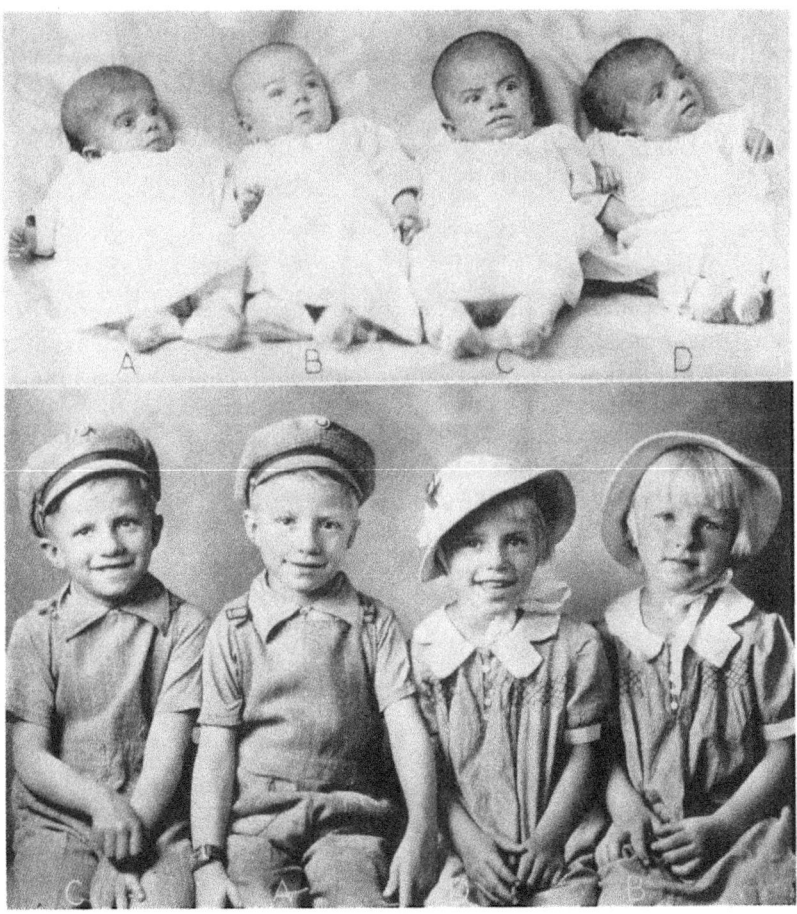

The **Schense** quads: *above,* aged 4½ months; *below,* age 5 years
(A – James; B – Joan; C – Jay; D – Jean) (Pryor 1939)

considering their prematurity. Birthweights, in order of delivery, were approximately 1560, 2210, 1685 and 2040g. There were two boys and two girls. The single placenta was not examined for a diagnosis of zygosity. Pryor concluded from later radiographic analysis of their bone ossification patterns (see Chapter 5, pp. 51–52) that they were a TZ set, the two boys possibly being MZ twins.

The quads—Joan, Jean, James and Jay—left hospital at 7 weeks and progressed normally except for being slightly underweight. A psychological examination before school entry at 6 years showed normal intelligence for all four children. As the parents were having trouble making ends meet, the local community elected a 'Schense Quadruplet Control Committee' to promote the general welfare of the children (see Chapter 4, p. 37).

In reporting on the set at 13 years (see Table 5.III, p. 50), Gardner and Newman (1944) disagreed with Pryor's original zygosity determination and described them as a QZ set who 'are in no way different from four siblings except that they are of the same age.' They concluded:

It appears that we were wrong in our original opinion that the ovulation of four eggs at once, their successful fertilization, implantation and placentation, gestation, birth and survival as healthy individuals, was a highly improbable event. As a matter of fact, four-egg quadruplets seem to be commoner than any other zygotic type.

Gardner, I.C., Newman, H.H. (1944) 'Studies of quadruplets. VII—The Schenses, four-egg quadruplets.' *Journal of Heredity*, **35**, 83–88.
Pryor, J.W. (1939) 'Normal variations in the ossification of bones due to genetic factors.' *Journal of Heredity*, **30**, 249–255.

ANON., *9 March 1931—none surviving.*

For the 23-year-old mother, this was her first pregnancy. In the second or third month she sought an abortion, but this was refused because she appeared to be around three-and-a-half months pregnant. Four months later she was attended by a midwife who delivered a girl of 6 months gestational age. When the placenta had not arrived an hour later the midwife sent the mother to hospital. Within minutes a boy was born. An hour and a half later, in place of the awaited placenta, two more babies were born, both boys. All the children were born alive but none lived longer than 90 minutes. The total weight was 4940g. In his account of the birth, Dobis (1936) suggested they were a DZ set, the boys being MZ 'triplets', but the evidence provided was not conclusive.

Dobis, A.G. (1936) 'Grossesse terminée par la naissance de quatre foetus.' *Gynécologie et Obstétrique*, **33**, 517–519.

ANON., *20 March 1931—none surviving.*

This is the first recorded instance of a quadruplet pregnancy being diagnosed by abdominal X-ray. The babies—two girls and two boys—were born at around seven to eight months gestation after a slow, uneventful labour. All died within three hours of delivery.

Hermstein, A., Pfalz, G.J. (1931) 'Eingeheude röntgenographische und geburtshilfe Beobachtung einer Vierlingsschwangerschaft und -geburt.' *Muenchener Medizinische Wochenschrift*, **78**, 492–496.

Pfalz, G.J. (1931) 'Röntgendiagnose einer Vierlingsschwangerschaft.' *Röntgenpraxis*, **3**, 328–332.

ANON., *South Cameroons, late-1932—three surviving at 3½ years.*
The mother belonged to a Pygmy tribe living in forestland just north of the Equator. Her age was estimated at around 25 to 30 years and she had one daughter of 12 or 13 years. Not much was known about the circumstances of her confinement except that it was 'a day of great effort', and the birth was assisted by the women of the tribe. The first to be delivered was a boy who, though he showed signs of life, died shortly after birth. Three live daughters followed, who resembled each other to the extent that they were often confused. They remained in good health, apart from an ulcer that needed treatment. In the medical report, Nicolle (1935) pointed out that, unlike the celebrated Dionnes, this mother and her daughters did not have the benefit of obstetrical or medical assistance. They survived in an environment of tropical diseases, and were nourished for 15 months by their mother's milk only. Nicolle was not able to meet the father of the family and could not follow the development of the children because of the Pygmy way of life.

Nicolle, G. (1935) 'A propos d'un cas de fécondité quadri-gémellaire chez une femme de race pygmée.' *Bulletin de la Société d'Obstétrique et de Gynécologie*, **24**, 611–614.

ANON., *USA, 15 April 1933—none surviving.*
This all-girl set was born near Yale University. It was the mother's 11th pregnancy, and she had previously had seven normal births—two of twins—and three miscarriages. Birth occurred at a gestational age of 5½ months calculated from the mother's last menstrual period. She entered hospital in the second stage of labour and the babies were delivered within the next 30 minutes. All were born alive, but none survived more than 1 hour. The dead infants were preserved but not the placentae. A very thorough study of the infants was made, including a full anthropometric record, anatomical studies and X-ray examination of the skeletons. Analysis of foot and hand prints suggested that they were a DZ set comprising two pairs of MZ 'twins', but there was no analysis of the birth membranes from which to check this conclusion.

Diddle, A.W., Burford, T.H. (1935) 'A study of a set of quadruplets.' *Anatomical Record*, **61**, 281–293.

ANON., *14 May 1934—three surviving.*
A report of this birth was made by the midwife and remained unchecked by any medical officer. The mother was 23 years old and had one previous child. The quads were diagnosed by X-ray. Labour began one week before term; the first stage was painless and of unknown length, the second stage lasted three hours 12 minutes and the third stage, 18 minutes. The mother 'delivered herself rapidly of four living male children'. The total weight was 7655g. The largest child died the next day but the other three did well.

Lloyd, B. (1934) 'Obstetrical rarities.' *British Medical Journal*, **1**, 1089.

GALE, *USA, reported 1935—all surviving.*
A note in the *Journal of Heredity*, appended to a brief report on the Derner quadruplets, mentioned this all-girl set who apparently were monozygotic and 'lived to maturity'. However, no further details were given and no other reports could be located.

Journal of Heredity (1935) 'The Derner quadruplets.' **26**, 256.

JOHNSON, *New Zealand, 6 March 1935—all surviving.*
These quads were the first surviving set in New Zealand. They were born in Dunedin, a city with a University Medical School and a specialist Infants' Hospital. The mother was 34 years old and had had three previous deliveries of single infants, one of whom had died on the third day after birth. She was admitted to hospital, unaware of the multiple gestation, in her seventh month of pregnancy. An X-ray showed three fetal heads and four vertebral columns. Nine days after admission labour began spontaneously. About two hours later the first baby was born, a boy

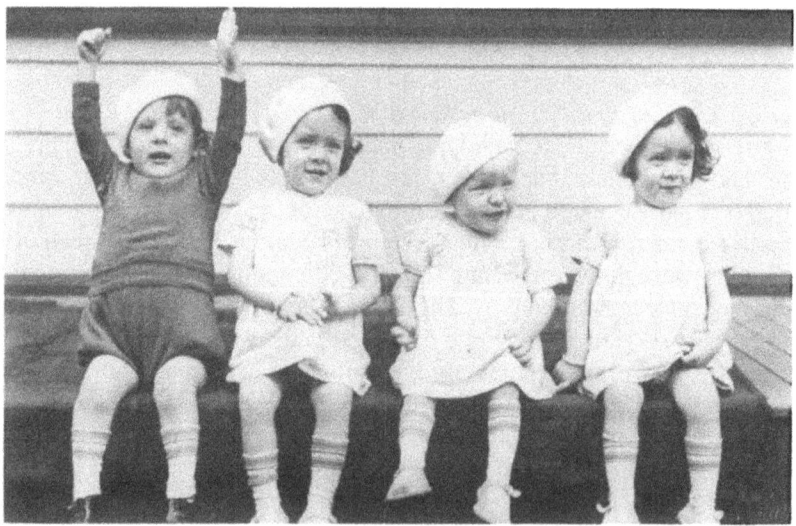

The **Johnson** quads (from the personal collection of Mrs Catherine Johnson)

weighing about 2100g. It was a further four hours until the delivery of the next child, a girl of 1955g. In another 30 minutes a second girl was born, weighing 1785g, and the last girl arrived 30 minutes later, weighing 2070g. The labour lasted a total of seven hours 15 minutes, and was uncomplicated except for some uterine inertia and the tedious delay between the arrival of the first and second babies. Examination of the placentae suggested that this was a TZ conception, the second and third born being MZ twins.

Details of the birth, the feeding and nursing regimes, and the infants' subsequent development were reported by Dawson (1936). At 3 days the quads (named Bruce, Kathleen, Mary and Vera) were transferred to the Truby-King Infant Hospital. The mother joined them there two weeks later, staying with them for a month during which time two were partially breast-fed. At 6 months the quads' progress was satisfactory. Prints from hands and feet were found to differ (casting some doubt on the original zygosity determination), and blood types (not specified) were identical, being the same as the parents'. The children were kept in the Infants' Hospital until they were 10½ months old. As they grew up, the 'twin pair' remained hard to tell apart—according to the mother, both the father and the girls' various boyfriends had had problems with this (*personal communication*). At the time of writing they are 54 years of age, all living. One girl has been in a home for the retarded since the age of 12. The others are all married with families—including one set of twins—and one is a grandparent.

The mother, Mrs Catherine Johnson, aged 81 at the time these notes were compiled, added an interesting comment on her family history. Her mother's maiden name was Wroblenski and her grandparents came to New Zealand from Poland. Her great uncle remembered a family funeral in Poland, which he recounted to her. It took place sometime between 1830 and 1870, at a big church. Four white coffins were laid out with four babies in them. It was assumed that they had been a quadruplet set.

The mother lived to the age of 82. She died on 4 August 1983, survived by her four famous children.

Dawson, J.B. (1936) 'A case of quadruplets.' *Journal of Obstetrics and Gynaecology of the British Empire*, **43**, 252–266.

Department of Pathology, Medical School, University of Otago, New Zealand (1935) *Daybook Registration (DB 6/2618), 7th March. Specimen of Multiple Placenta Pregnancy (4).*

ANON., *Netherlands, 9 July 1935—two stillborn, two surviving at 5 weeks.*
The mother, who lived in Utrecht, was aged 31 years and had had three previous pregnancies, all uneventful. Her sister had one set of twins. The quadruplet gestation was not diagnosed until after the birth of the first child. Labour commenced at 6.30am. The membranes ruptured spontaneously with little discharge of amniotic fluid. The first child was born at 10.15am and two more followed minutes later. The fourth baby was delivered after the membranes of its separate amniotic sac were ruptured. This was an all-girl set, and the second and fourth were stillborn. The birthweights of the first and third babies were 1600 and 1750g respectively; the dead infants were not weighed. The two survivors progressed well and at 5 weeks were reported to be in good health. The quads were thought to be an MZ set.

Frijda, L.J. (1935) 'Casuistische Mededeelingen: Een eeneiige Vierling.' *Nederlandsch Tijdschrift voor Geneeskunde*, **79**, 4896–4898.

ANON., *England, 12–13 October 1935—two surviving as infants.*
The mother, aged 34 years, had had three previous pregnancies. In the seventh month a skiagram indicated quadruplets. An X-ray taken one month before the

birth placed the gestational age at 34 weeks; it was further predicted that they were all boys. Though somewhat hazardous, this prediction proved correct. Labour began spontaneously and the first child was delivered by forceps. The second baby arrived 25 minutes later, the third within another 15 minutes and the fourth 10 minutes after that. Birthweights ranged from 950 to 1645g. The first and second babies, who were MZ 'twins' with a single amniotic sac, died at 3 and 6 days. The third and fourth had separate placentae, and were still living at the time the cases were reported.

Constantine, M.C.E. (1935) 'A case of quadruplets.' *British Medical Journal*, **2**, 1206–1207.
Williams, E.U. (1935) 'Ante-natal diagnosis of quadruplets.' *British Medical Journal*, **2**, 1206.

MILES, *England, 28 November 1935—all surviving.*
The Miles quads were the first (reported) surviving set in the British Isles. The births occurred at Eynesbury, near St. Neots, in Huntingdonshire. (In reports, they are referred to alternatively as either the St. Neots quads or the Eynesbury quads.) The mother was aged 33 years and this was her second pregnancy. An X-ray at five months revealed three babies. She had at least two prenatal checks, and a home delivery at around 32 weeks. Dr Harrisson was called to her cottage when the waters broke at 1.30am and the first child, a girl, was born without assistance at 3.18am. The doctor ruptured the membranes for the next two babies—both boys—the first arriving at 3.47am and the second at 5.06am. Chloroform was used for the first time before delivery of the fourth child, another boy, at 5.44am. This last baby needed help to establish breathing. The birthweights ranged from 1275 to 1785g. The afterbirth, which was preserved in the museum of the Bedford County Hospital, comprised a large central twin placenta with two smaller placentae attached to it on either side with no connecting vessels. The large placenta was symmetrical and showed no division; there were two distinct amniotic sacs, but the partition was only partial. It was concluded that the quads were a TZ set.

Because it was impossible to maintain an even temperature in the parent's house, the doctor moved the children to his own home (see Chapter 1, p. 3). The services of four trained nurses from Great Ormond Street Hospital for Sick Children, London, were obtained. The quads' development during the first nine months of life was traced by Harrisson (1936), who revealed that the parents did not get to see their children again until Christmas Day, although the Gaumont British Film Company had started filming the quads the day before. The infants (named Ann, Ernest, Paul and Michael) moved to the parents' new home when they were 6 months old; a nursery ('a big airy room facing south') was added as an extension to the house. Three months later the doctor reported:

All four children are extremely well and happy. Their complexions are beautiful, their skins perfect . . . They are very intelligent, and quickly recognize their friends. They can pull themselves up, and can roll over by themselves in their cribs. They sleep the whole night through without a murmur, and might easily be taken for the babies of four different confinements instead of quadruplets prematurely born.

Harrisson, E.H. (1935) 'The Eynesbury quadruplets.' *British Medical Journal*, **2**, 1207–1208.
—— (1936) 'The Eynesbury quadruplets. First nine months of life.' *British Medical Journal*, **2**, 917–920.

WYCOFF, *USA, reported 1936—all surviving.*
This set—one male and three females, living in Sac City, IA—is mentioned by Pryor (1936) in a report on the ossification of bones in the hands of quadruplets. X-rays were taken at 1 year 4 months but 'the attending physician . . . was taken sick shortly after sending me the films and I am unable to give a full report.' Pryor stated that 'I will make a full report some time in the future'; however, no such report could be located.

Pryor, J.W. (1936) 'Ossification as additional evidence in differentiating identicals and fraternals in multiple births.' *American Journal of Anatomy*, **59**, 409–423.

KASPAR, *USA, 9 May 1936—all surviving.*
The family circumstances of this set have been detailed in Chapter 4 (p. 38). The first of the quads to be delivered was a girl, birthweight approximately 1675g, and was named Frances. There followed three boys: Frank (1701g), Felix (1276g) and Ferdinand (1644g).

Dr Iva Gardner studied the quads at 4 years 3 months, and her findings were reported in the fifth of her and H.H. Newman's 'Studies of quadruplets' in the

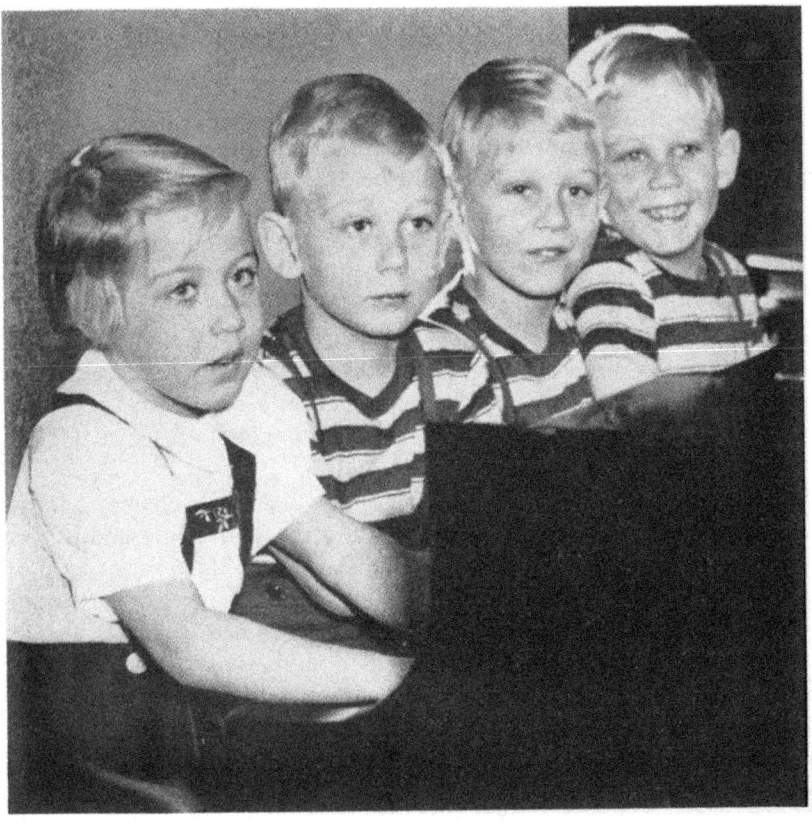

The **Kaspar** quads (Gardner and Newman 1943)

Journal of Heredity. No information had been recorded regarding the placentae; however, based on dermatoglyphic evidence from the quads' palm- and fingerprints, they were diagnosed as a DZ set comprising MZ male 'triplets' and a female 'sibling'.

[The palmprints] would, in the absence of any other data, afford conclusive evidence that the set is a two-egg set . . . This diagnosis would be strongly reinforced by a study of the physical correspondences of the three boys [who] are all as similar to one another as the average pair of one-egg twins, but Felix and Ferdinand are so extremely similar that even their mother has difficulty in distinguishing them. Frank is only a little less similar to the two other boys, but as much like them as one-egg twins usually are like each other. All of the quads are described by Dr. Gardner as "the sturdiest, huskiest set of quads I have ever seen."

Without any knowledge of the placental relations, we can only guess at the embryonic history of this set of quadruplets. Our guess is that the first of the two zygotes to reach the uterus and to become implanted was the Frances zygote, that the second zygote was delayed in implantation and as a consequence underwent an early division into twin primordia, and that later one of these twin primordia divided again to form a secondary pair of twins. Since mirror imaging is strongest between Ferdinand and Felix it is our guess that these two are the product of the later twinning division.

Gardner, I.C., Newman, H.H. (1943) 'Studies of quadruplets. V—the Kaspar quadruplets.' *Journal of Heredity*, **34**, 27–32.

ANON., *England, 12 June 1938—one surviving.*
The mother had had four previous pregnancies; her age is not stated. She first attended the antenatal clinic at Walton Hospital, Liverpool, when she was 25 weeks pregnant but the uterus was as it would be at 38 weeks in a normal pregnancy. Multiple status was suspected and quadruplets were confirmed by X-ray. She was admitted to hospital at 29 weeks and labour began spontaneously a month later. Preparations had been made in advance and a colour film was made of the birth—possibly the first use of this approach in the documentation of a multiple birth. (The film was subsequently shown at the Royal Society of Medicine.) The four babies were delivered within a space of 15 minutes, all by breech presentation. The afterbirth was delivered complete: the placenta of the first child was quite separate from those of the others, which were completely fused together. It was concluded that they were a QZ set.

The first child, a boy weighing 1445g (and named William), cried well on delivery, but on the following two days had attacks of cyanosis and died. The second baby, a girl of 2210g (Veronica), also had attacks of cyanosis but subsequently recovered and was still alive at the time the report was made. The third infant, a boy of 1870g (Bryan), needed assistance to establish breathing, and had cyanosis and twitching which subsided on the second day. He survived to 4 months, dying then of pneumonia. The last to be delivered was a boy of 1815g (Alan); he suffered asphyxia at birth, became cyanosed the next day, started convulsions at 11 days and died at 13 days of cerebral haemorrhage.

Wilson, St. G. (1939) 'The birth of quadruplets.' *Proceedings of the Royal Society of Medicine*, **32** (Obstetrical and Gynaecological Section), 1220–1222.

BADGETT, *USA, 1 February 1939—all surviving.*
The parents, who lived in Galveston, TX, already had two daughters, of 13 and 15 years, when these quads were born. By dates they were five to six weeks preterm. X-ray had shown only three skeletons and the presence of the fourth was not suspected. Spontaneous rupture of one amnion precipitated delivery which was normal and brief. The set comprised four girls, two with blue eyes and two with brown eyes. One child (Joan) was attached to a single placenta; she was the heaviest (at 2085g) and learned to walk first. The other three (Jeanette, Jeraldine, Joyce) all weighed between 1750 and 1760g; they had a common placenta but there were two chorionic sacs attached to it. Sinclair (1940) concluded that they were a TZ set, comprising one pair of MZ and one pair of DZ 'twins'. Gardner and Newman (1942), however, argued that it was not inconsistent with the placental evidence that the three babies attached to the large placenta were monozygotic even though there were two chorions.

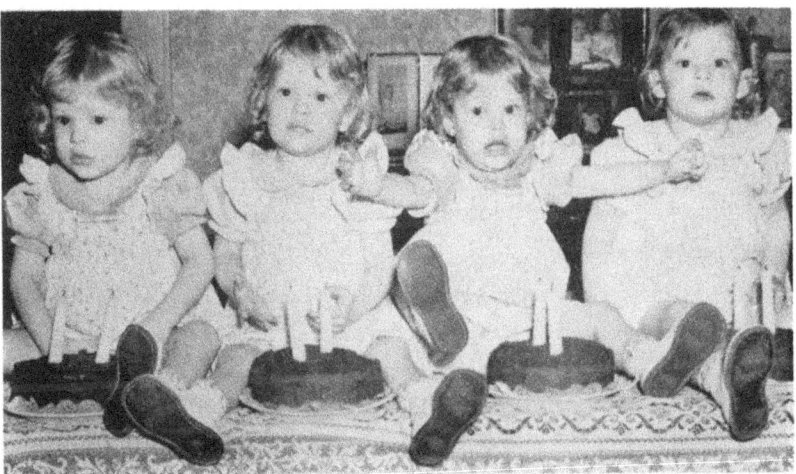

The **Badgett** quads on their second birthday (*l–r*, Jeraldine, Jeannette, Joyce, Joan)
(Gardner and Newman 1942)

The birth received a great amount of publicity (see Chapter 1, p. 4). Sinclair (1940) considered that the 'unusual combination of identical and non-identical twins in the same quadruplet group and the fact that they will receive continuous study while being given unusual opportunities for development makes this a very fine test case for ideas concerning the influences of nature and nurture in ontogeny.' Physical characteristics at 1 year were reported by Gardner and Newman (see Table 5.III, p. 50); however, there are no developmental data in any subsequent reports.

Gardner, I.C., Newman, H.H. (1942) 'Studies of quadruplets. IV—the Badgett quadruplets.' *Journal of Heredity*, **33**, 345–350.
Sinclair, J.G. (1940) 'The Badgett quadruplets.' *Journal of Heredity*, **31**, 163–164.

ANON., *USA, c.1940—miscarried.*
The 26-year-old mother, who lived in Winston, Salem, NC, had had three previous pregnancies, resulting in two singleton births and one set of twins. The miscarriage occurred at the 17th week. The placentae are pictured in the report, with the fetuses attached. Two girls each had a separate placenta, and a girl and a boy were attached to two fused placentae. The walls between these two were dissected, revealing two amniotic sacs and two chorionic sacs, which were not fused. This was a QZ set.

Miller, R.E. (1941) 'Quadruplets.' *Anatomical Record*, **80**, 411–420.

ANON., *USA, 6 February 1941—all surviving.*
The mother was 37 years old and lived in Fargo, ND. She presented herself for examination at about the sixth month of pregnancy according to her dates. An X-ray revealed four heads and she was hospitalized. The onset of labour was spontaneous (the timing in weeks is not given). Delivery was quick—total time was less than five minutes—and uneventful, the mother receiving a minimum of analgesia. First born was a girl, followed by three boys. Birthweights ranged from 1700 to 2100g. The girl was from a separate amniotic sac and was of group B blood type; the three boys were all group O and were considered to be MZ triplets. However, there was no satisfactory description of the birth membranes in the report. Growth and development to 2 years was described, including charts of the infants' heights and weights. Photographs at 2 years suggested that their general development was normal.

Lancaster, W.E.G. (1944) 'Growth and development of premature quadruplets.' *Journal—Lancet*, **64**, 147–152.

LASHLEY, *USA, 23 February 1941—all surviving.*
This family lived in Leitchfield, KY. The mother, who already had eight children, was in her seventh month of pregnancy when labour began. She gave birth to the first baby, a girl, without medical assistance. The family physician was summoned and the other three infants—a girl, a boy and a third girl—were delivered at intervals of two hours, one hour 45 minutes and 15 minutes. Birthweights ranged from 1615 to 2185g. An incubator was secured and the boy was placed in it as he appeared the weakest. 'The three girls were wrapped in blankets, warmed with hot water bottles, and placed in rocking chairs before a grate fire.' Later an ambulance was summoned to take them to the Louisville City Hospital. The girls were found to be in good condition; the boy suffered marked respiratory distress but responded well to treatment. No blood or membrane analysis was conducted, but studies of their physical characteristics suggested that they were a TZ set. They were named Beulah, Martine, John and Mildred. Their subsequent progress to 2 years was excellent and the medical report made at that time stated that they 'have been remarkably free of infection, and gastrointestinal upsets have been rare, indeed.'

Bruce, J.W., Scott, E.P. (1944) 'The Lashley quadruplets.' *Journal of Pediatrics*, **25**, 447–453.

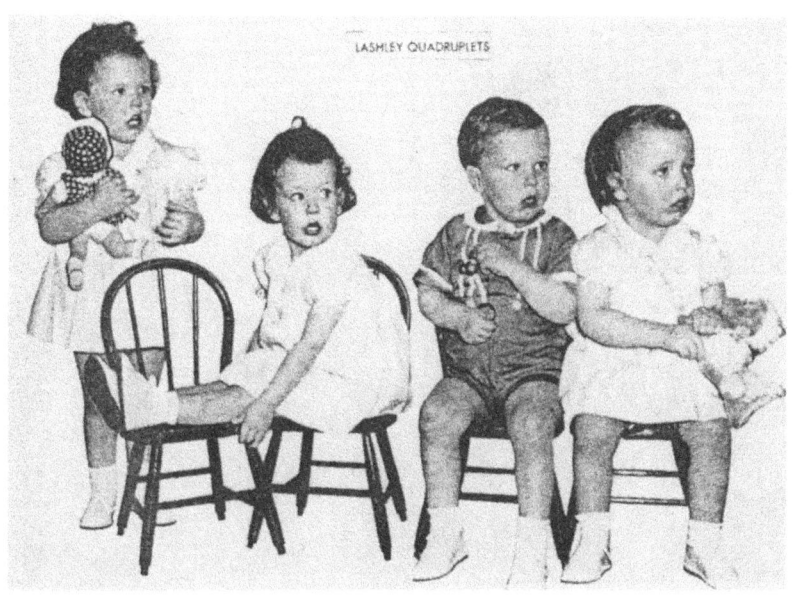

The **Lashley** quads (*l–r,* Mildred, Beulah, John, Martine) (Bruce and Scott 1944)

MENDOZA, *Venezuela, 3 April 1942—all surviving.*
The parents lived in a village high up in the Andes with a narrow track as the only access. The mother and infants survived the rigours of the first few days in difficult conditions. The mother, who was aged 30, had had three children, including twins from a previous marriage. The pregnancy was trouble-free and apparently went to full term as birth occurred at the time the mother had expected it. Labour commenced on the 2nd April and the first child was delivered at 11am on the 3rd April, the others following soon after. There were two boys and two girls, all in good health. The midwife reported that there was one placenta with four cords, but this was not available for examination. They are reported as being either a DZ or QZ set.

On the second day after the birth a doctor who happened to be in the vicinity examined the quads and arranged with the regional government for their transfer to the nearest hospital. On admission the two boys and two girls weighed 1980, 1375, 1305 and 1235g respectively. They remained in hospital and progressed well for the two months up to the time of the first report. A committee was formed to oversee their care and welfare.

Zubillaga, A., González, L.Z. (1942) 'Primera comunicacion sobre los cuadruples Mendoza.' *Archivos Venezolanos de Puericultura y Pediatria*, **4**, 641–647.
—— (1943) 'Segunda comunicacion de los cuadruples Mendoza.' *Archivos Venezolanos de Puericultura y Pediatria*, **5**, 888–904.

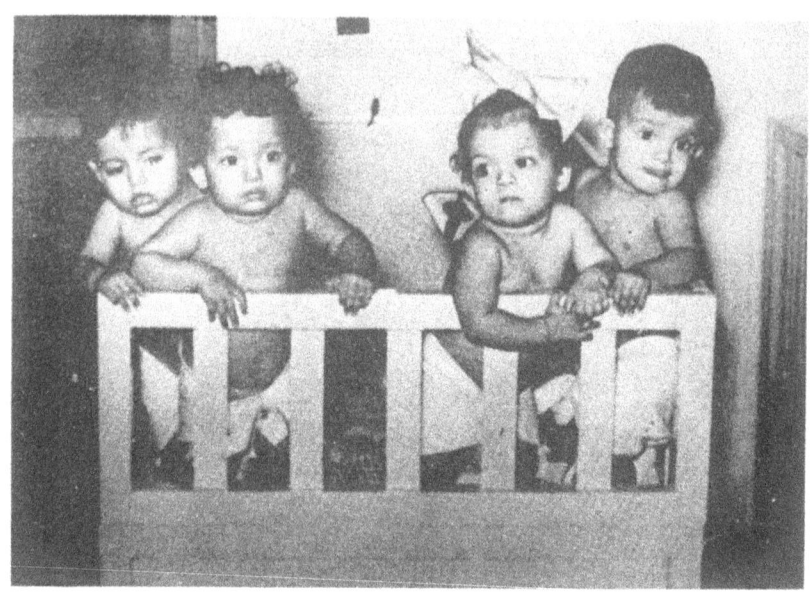

The **Mendoza** quads (Zubillaga 1943)

ANON., *France, 3 November 1943—none surviving beyond 3 months.*
The mother, who lived in Bannalec, Brittany, was 31 years old and already had three children. At six months her size suggested a multiple pregnancy. At seven months an X-ray showed three heads with the possibility of a fourth. The birth was by forceps delivery—two girls, both weighing 1475g, followed by two boys of 1700 and 1875g. The girls were attached to a single placenta with communicating blood vessels, while the boys had separate placentae. The girls were stated to be monozygotic, although no blood group analysis or dermatoglyphic study was done. The parents could not have all four babies at home so two were placed in a crèche. One boy and one girl died within a few days and neither of the others survived beyond 3 months.

Lartigue and Prudent (1944) 'Les quadruplées de Bannalec.' *Gynécologie et Obstétrique*, **44**, 23–24.

ZARIEF, *USA, 29 March 1944—all surviving.*
The mother was 27 years old and lived in New York. She had had two previous pregnancies, the first being terminated at an early stage, the second resulting in a live birth. She consulted her doctor at 14½ weeks and the size of her uterus suggested the probability of a multiple pregnancy. At four-and-a-half months she was admitted to hospital for a few days bed-rest, being then the size of a mother at full term with a singleton pregnancy. An X-ray at that time revealed four fetuses. She was re-admitted in her 27th week and confined to bed until she went into

spontaneous labour in her 35th week. The fetal heart rates, taken in the last month of pregnancy, varied considerably and did not show any constant relationship with each other. According to the report by Watson (1945) the ease of labour was noteworthy, lasting seven-and-a-half hours. The babies were born at about 10-minute intervals. Uterine tone was fairly good throughout, increasing as each successive baby was born. There were three girls and a boy; birthweights ranged from 2160 to 2270g. Analysis of the placentae and membranes, and microscopic analysis of the placental tissue (amnion, chorion, chorion, amnion) suggested QZ status. At 7 months the infants (Isodora, Ellen, Elaine and Benjamin) were easily distinguished from one another. Walker (1947) confirmed the QZ diagnosis by means of palm- and footprints; she also reported differences in the timing of the eruption of teeth.

Walker, N.F. (1947) 'A further description of a set of quadriovular quadruplets. (A study of dermal configurations and tooth eruption.)' *American Journal of Obstetrics and Gynecology*, **54**, 266–272.
Watson, B.P. (1945) 'A quadriovular quadruplet pregnancy.' *American Journal of Obstetrics and Gynecology*, **50**, 184–190.

ANON., *USA, 1 November 1944—all surviving at 1 month.*
The mother (Mrs K.C.) lived in Philadelphia, PA. Her first pregnancy had resulted in the delivery of a stillborn baby by caesarian section two weeks before term. By the fifth month of this multiple pregnancy she was large for dates; X-ray revealed four fetuses and she was immediately hospitalized. At seven months she had irregular contractions and because of her previous history it was decided to perform a caesarian section to avoid possible rupture of the uterus. One placenta was on the outer wall and it was necessary to go through it to reach the babies. According to the report, the first three infants delivered 'were all female babies and were enclosed in a single sac' (it is not clear whether this refers to an amnion or chorion), while the fourth, a boy, 'was in a separate amnion with a small separate placenta'. Birthweights ranged from 1304 to 1758g. The babies were kept in an incubator for the first month of life.

Ullery, J.C. (1945) 'Delivery of quadruplets by cesarian section under continuous spinal anaesthesia.' *Journal of the American Medical Association*, **128**, 183–185.

HENN, *USA, 23 December 1946—all surviving at 4 months.*
The mother, who lived in Baltimore, MD, was 26 years old and had one child already. There was no history of multiple birth in her family or her husband's. She presented herself to the obstetrician at around three to three-and-a-half months. Nothing unusual was found, except that the size of the uterus indicated a birth in December rather than the following February as had been predicted. It was assumed that the mother had erred in her dates. At six months two fetal heartbeats were heard. X-ray examination on November 18th revealed a quadruplet pregnancy. Onset of labour was spontaneous at 235 days (menstrual age), and birth occurred by vaginal delivery without anaesthesia and with no serious pain. The babies—three boys and one girl—were born 10 to 30 minutes apart. An unusual

aspect of this delivery was the delivery of the first placenta following the first baby and before the subsequent babies. The second placenta was delivered as a fused mass after the other three babies. An indiscreet mention to a reporter of the possibility that these three were an identical triplet group gave rise to inaccurate newspaper reports which were widely circulated. In fact the placentae and membranes indicated that the quads were a QZ set, the three fused membranes

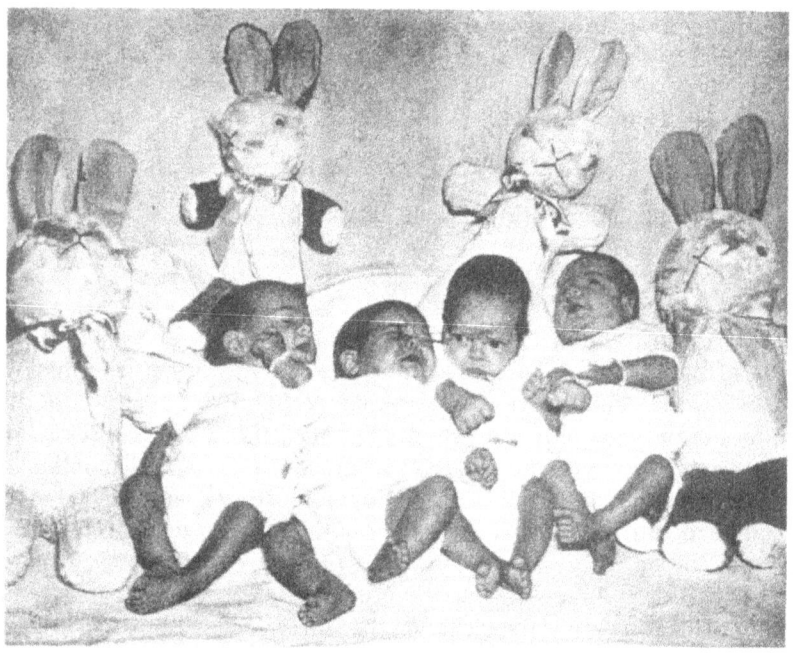

The **Henn** quads (Gedda 1951)

being separated by both chorionic and amniotic membranes. Birthweights were from 1320 to 1920g. The infants thrived under paediatric care up to the last report at 4 months. The photograph above is reproduced from Gedda's comprehensive anthology of twin studies, *Studio dei Gemelli*.

Bowyer, T.S., Corner, G.W. (1947) 'Premature quadruplets.' *American Journal of Obstetrics and Gynecology*, **54**, 1033–1037.
Gedda, L. (1951) *Studio dei Gemelli*. Rome: Edizioni Orizzonte Medico (p. 165).

ANON. c.*1946–1948, no birth details—all surviving at 12 years.*
Scott (1960) reported the psychological examination of a quad set at 12 years. There were two boys and two girls. The report is limited to interpretation of the test results; no other details of the quads were given and it has not been possible to match this set with a corresponding birth report in the literature. The quads had been placed in a foster home, having lived in a disturbed family setting and

following the divorce of the parents. WISC Full-scale intelligence scores were 70, 72, 77 and 79. Rorschach and Thematic Apperception tests were administered and interpreted. The author stated that this was the only known report of psychological test results for quadruplets at that time. This claim was not in fact true, but may be indicative of the difficulty of locating material on these rare groups.

Scott, E.M. (1960) 'Psychological examination of quadruplets.' *Psychological Reports*, **6**, 281–282.

ANON., *USSR, 7 October 1947—all surviving.*
The 35-year-old mother had had nine previous pregnancies all of which had ended in abortion. In the eighth month she was admitted to Tokmaksaya Hospital, Kurgizia, in good health. Vaginal delivery occurred an hour later. The quads, all boys, were born about an hour apart, the total delivery time being around five hours. Birthweights were approximately 1400, 1500, 1500 and 1700g. There were three placentae; one was large and typical of the structure found in MZ twins.

Demba, Z.A. (1952) 'Birth with four fetuses.' *Akusherstvo i Ginekologiya*, **3**, 73.

ZAVADA, *USA, 14 February 1948—all surviving.*
Hartman *et al.* (1949) reported this case as the earliest positive diagnosis of quads on record, seen on X-ray at 17 weeks. The mother was 25 years old and lived in Latrobe, PA. At 31 weeks one boy and three girls were delivered by caesarian section, obviously preterm, and each weighing slightly over 1360g. The boy was from a single, separate placenta and the girls from a large common placenta with separate amniotic sacs and a single chorion. A reference to paediatric consultations suggests that the children survived and developed well, but it was not possible to trace this case any further. A photograph of the quads appears in Gedda's *Studio dei Gemelli*.

Gedda, L. (1951) *Studio dei Gemelli*. Rome: Edizioni Orizzonte Medico (p. 161).
Hartman, J.W., Feightner, F., Titus, P. (1949) 'Quadruplet pregnancy: diagnosis at seventeen weeks of gestation.' *American Journal of Obstetrics and Gynecology*, **57**, 1005–1007.

GOOD, *England, 12 June 1948—all surviving to adulthood.*
This set are referred to in reports as the 'Bristol quadruplets'. The mother was 27 years old with one daughter. At five months' gestation her abdominal enlargement was 'unusually great' but an X-ray showed only one fetus. At eight months she was admitted to Southmead Hospital, Bristol, and X-ray then clearly showed four fetal heads. The next day, due to rapid onset of toxaemia, a caesarian section was performed; there were no unusual problems and the patient made a rapid recovery. The babies, four girls weighing from 1730 to 2040g, made good progress. From analysis of the birth membranes—three placentae fused in one large mass—it was inferred that they were a TZ set. Their blood groups, checked for five components, were the same. They remained in hospital for three months while the local authority prepared a new home 'with electricity, and all modern facilities' for the

family. They were named Bridget, Jennifer, Elizabeth and Frances, and the latter pair were thought to be MZ 'twins'.

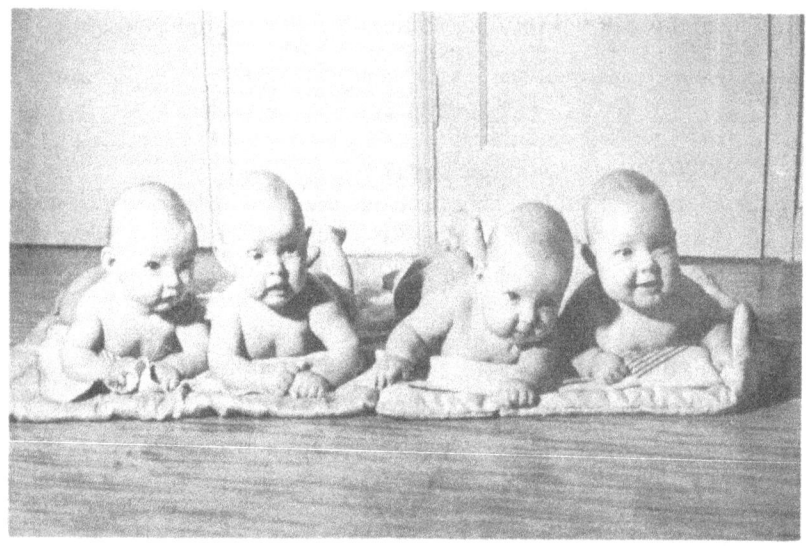

The **Good** quads (*l–r,* Jennifer, Bridget, Frances, Elizabeth)
(Shepherd and Potter 1949)

These quads are unique in that their normal development to 24 years of age has been reported. Their progress through school is outlined in Chapter 5 (p. 67); their physical growth records at birth, 1 year and 21 years are shown in Table 5.IV (p. 51); and their developmental outcomes and marital and vocational histories are detailed in Chapter 4 (p. 45). Similarities and differences within the set are consistent with the assumption of TZ status. For instance, the onset of menarche occurred within a month for the MZ pair (11:4 and 11:5), but earlier and later by several months for the other two sisters (10:6 and 11:8).

Corner, B.D. (1949) 'The quadruplets: 2. Management.' *Bristol Medico-Chirurgical Journal,* **66**, 14–16.
—— (1974) 'The Bristol quadruplets: Twenty-four year history.' *Acta Geneticae Medicae et Gemellologiae,* **22** (Suppl.), 149–153.
Shepherd, H.L., Potter, M.F. (1949) 'The quadruplets: 1. Delivery.' *Bristol Medico-Chirurgical Journal,* **66**, 14.
Watson-Williams, E.J. (1949) 'The quadruplets: 3. Notes.' *Bristol Medico-Chirurgical Journal,* **66**, 17–19.

ANON., *France, 5 September 1948—all surviving.*
The mother was 42 years old and had four surviving children from eight previous pregnancies. X-ray examination at eight months revealed the presence of four fetuses. Labour began spontaneously two weeks later. Two babies were born spontaneously within an hour, and two more after the administration of

chloroform. The birth order was boy, girl, boy, girl, and the birthweights ranged from 1750 to 2590g. Blood tests and analysis of the three placentae and birth membranes suggested TZ status, with the two boys being MZ twins. The case was reported to the Société de Pédiatrie de Paris on 26 April 1949, when the quads were said to be developing successfully.

Blechmann, G., Vaudescal, R., Levesque, A., Forestler, G. (1950) 'Note sûr les premiers jours des quadruples de la Celle-Saint-Cloud.' *Société de Pédiatrie de Paris*, 28 February, 612–613.
—— Joron, M., Joron, F. (1950) 'Note sûr l'élevage des quadruples.' *Société de Pédiatrie de Paris*, 28 February, 613–615.
Vaudescal, M.M., Blechmann, G., Levesque, A. (1948) 'Grossesse quadrigémellaire.' *Gynécologie et Obstétrique*, **47**, 883–887.

TAYLOR, *England, 21 September 1948—all surviving.*
The photograph below is reproduced from Gedda's *Studio dei Gemelli*. The brief caption stated that these quads—three boys and a girl—were born at the North Middlesex Hospital, London. No written report could be located; however, it

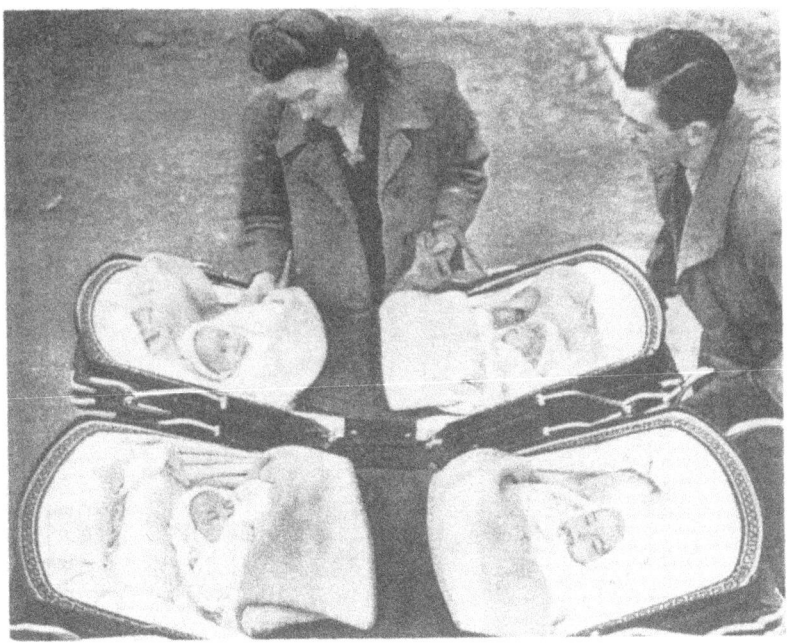

The **Taylor** quads (Gedda 1951)

seems probable that this is the set referred to in the table reproduced overleaf (from a review by McKeown and Record 1952), with the given birthdate of 21 *October* 1948, a simple mistake having been made concerning the month of birth.

Gedda, L. (1951) *Studio dei Gemelli*. Rome: Edizioni Orizzonte Medico (p. 139).

QUADRUPLET MATERNITIES IN ENGLAND AND WALES, 1931–1951, NOT INCLUDED ELSEWHERE IN THIS CATALOGUE*

LMP = date of first day of last menstrual period; EDC = expected date of confinement; L = liveborn; S = stillborn; D = died.

Date of delivery	Duration of gestation (weeks)	Method of estimation	Maternal age (years)	Parity	Fetus 1			Fetus 2			Fetus 3			Fetus 4		
					Sex	Weight (g)	Fate	Sex	Weight (g)	Fate	Sex	Weight (g)	Fate	Sex	Weight (g)	Fate
10.08.32	32	LMP early January 1932	30	6	F	1050	L	F	1135	L	M	1415	D	M	1390	D
29.11.34	31–35	EDC January 1935	35	6	M	1275	D	M	1190	D	M	1190	D	F	1105	D
28.03.37	35	LMP 22.07.36	38	3	M	1930	D	F	625	S	F	2070	L	F	2270	L
8.08.37	c.32	Delivery two months before expected date	26	1	M	1360	D	M	1360	L	M	1415	L	M	1445	D
4.11.37	31–35	LMP March 1937	31	3	F	1330	D	M	905	D	M	905	D	F	1275	D
8.03.40	32	LMP end July 1939	33	2	M	935	D	M	935	D	F	935	D	M	680	D
21.04.43	36	LMP 7.08.42	29	1	M	1135	S	M	1135	S	F	1815	L	F	1360	S
1.06.43	37	LMP 15.09.42	41	3	M	1360	D	M	1360	D	F	1360	D	F	1360	D
10.10.43	35	Delivery five weeks before expected date	28	2	F	1475	D	F	1245	S	F	1135	S	F	1560	L
28.02.44	c.31	LMP seven calendar months before birth	23	1	F	1700	L	F	1590	L	M	1590	L	M	1360	D
22.05.44	30	EDC 25.07.44	38	6	M	1545	L	M	835	D	F	1305	L	M	1530	L
3.06.44	33	LMP 13.10.43	31	3	F	1615	D	M	1730	D	F	1645	L	F	1415	L
8.12.44	34	LMP 10.04.44	23	1	F	1360	L	F	1530	D	F	1645	L	F	935	L
7.01.47	29	LMP 15.06.46	29	6	F	765	D	F	935	D	M	1020	D	M	1075	D
19.04.47	33	LMP 30.08.46	38	1	M	1360	L	F	905	D	M	795	D	F	820	D
22.08.47	27	LMP 10.02.47	25	2	F	850	D	F	810	D	F	665	S	F	595	S
28.09.47	30–31	Clinical estimate (no menstrual period since preceding confinement)	29	3	F	1105	D	F	880	D	F	820	D	F	1105	D
12.10.47	32	LMP 25.02.47	27	1	F	1305	D	F	1330	L	F	820	D	M	1615	D
18.07.48	20	Clinical estimate	?	3	M	480	S	F	540	D	M	515	D	M	490	D
21.10.48**	34	EDC first week in December	27	3	F	1530	L	M	1490	L	M	1915	L	M	1345	L
9.01.51	34	LMP 16.05.50	34	2	M	1445	L	M	1250	S	M	1390	L	F	1890	L
11.07.51	32	LMP 29.11.50	36	4	M	1360	L	M	1760	L	M	1645	D	F	1615	L
20.08.51	34	LMP 24.12.50	27	2	M	1050	L	F	1160	L	M	1420	D	F	880	L

*Adapted from McKeown and Record (1952). Cases included in this table were collected in the first instance from reports in the medical literature or in the national press. They were subsequently verified, and birth details ascertained, by writing to the obstetrician who conducted the delivery (in the case of hospital confinements) or to the family's general practitioner (for home deliveries). Six cases have been omitted from the original table as details are already included elsewhere in this Catalogue.

**See entry for Taylor quads (21 September 1948).

POLZER, *Germany, c.1949—all surviving.*
Three girls and a boy, born in Gedern. The mother already had five other children. A photograph is reproduced in Gedda's *Studio dei Gemelli*, but no further details are given.

Gedda, L. (1951) *Studio dei Gemelli.* Rome: Edizioni Orizzonte Medico (p. 139).

ANON., *Australia, 17–19 August 1950—all surviving.*
The mother was 29 years old, lived in Bellingham, NSW, and had had one previous confinement. She was under medical supervision from the second month. By five months the size of the uterus suggested the possibility of a multiple pregnancy. By the sixth month multiparity was obvious but X-ray examination was delayed until 32 weeks. Three fetuses were shown on the film. Further X-rays 10 days later showed quads. From the eighth month the problem was whether or not to allow the fetuses to mature further while having to control the mother's toxaemia. From the report by Elliot *et al.* (1951) it appears that she was not admitted to hospital until the onset of labour. There was a severe degree of uterine inertia, the uterus giving up as soon as resistance to its efforts was encountered. The first baby, a girl of 1630g, was delivered after eight hours of labour; contractions then stopped for over two hours. The authors of the medical report stated that after 13 hours 'we were fortified by the condition of the mother and the foetus and decided against interference.' The second baby was delivered 26 hours after the first and was a boy of 2580g. After a further 17 hours the third baby was born (a girl, 2268g) and the fourth (a boy, 1673g) arrived seven-and-a-half hours after that. By virtue of their birth dates the babies differed in length of gestation—263 days for the first born, 264 days for the second and 265 days for the last two. There were two placental masses. The larger was composed of two placentae, one of which served a pair, probably the two girls, the other serving one of the boys. The smaller one came away last and was connected to the second boy.

At 6 months the four children were developing well and in good health. A study of their blood groups firmly established that they were a QZ set. This can be seen by taking the sex and ABO grouping, or the sex and MN groups, or by taking the ABO and MN groups together and disregarding sex. The tests were made using capillary blood.

Elliot, M.E.H., Hewitt, G.H., Elphinstone, K.R., Ostinga, A.J., Mayes, B.T. (1951) 'The birth of quadruplets: a successful case of pregnancy and confinement complicated by multiple pregnancy (quadruplets), preeclamptic toxemia and uterine inertia.' *Medical Journal of Australia*, **1**, 690–693.
Walsh, R.J. (1952) 'The blood groups of quadruplets.' *Australasian Annals of Medicine*, **1**, 140–141.

ANON., *England, 12–13 September 1950—all surviving to adulthood.*
The mother (Mrs M.C.) was 27 years old and already had one son. The pregnancy proceeded normally to the fifth month, no concern being felt about size because of doubts about the date of the mother's last menstrual period. Multiple pregnancy was first suspected in the sixth month, and a skiagram taken in the seventh month indicated 'at least' three fetuses. The radiologist requested a second exposure and

the presence of quads was confirmed on August 4th. Soon after, the mother was admitted to the Westminster Hospital, London, where preparations were made for the birth, including the installation of special incubators in a prepared room and a full-time team of trained nurses on stand-by. At 12.15am on 12th September the membranes ruptured; labour commenced 20½ hours later at 8.45pm and was uncomplicated, lasting in total just over three-and-a-half hours. All four babies were girls. The first two were born at 11.34pm and 11.48pm on 12th September, the third and fourth at 12.17am and 12.20am on 13th September. The third baby had difficulty establishing breathing but otherwise they were in good condition. Birthweights ranged from 1475 to 1785g. The placenta was very large and thick, and the birth membranes were described as being 'very ragged'. Sections of the membranes were taken between the sacs, the report stating that 'it is quite clear that all four sacs consist of amnion only, the whole being contained by a single chorion and therefore associated with a common placenta, i.e., the quadruplets are uniovular.' Preliminary blood group analysis showed that all four infants were group A, Rh+. (A second report was not located.) Follow-up at 1 year showed the quads to be developing normally.

The quads were featured in an article in the 8 July 1984 edition of *You* magazine (a colour supplement of the *Mail on Sunday* newspaper). The article recorded that the sisters—Edna, Frances, Marie and Patsy—were all married, three of them with children (none of them multiple births).

Searle, W.N., Denny, F. (1953) 'A case of uniovular quadruplets.' *Journal of Obstetrics and Gynaecology of the British Empire*, **60**, 31–36.

WALSER, *France, reported 1951—all liveborn.*
A picture of this all-girl set, born at the hospital of St. Louis of Parigi in Paris, appears in Gedda's *Studio dei Gemelli*. No further details are given.

Gedda, L. (1951) *Studio dei Gemelli.* Rome: Edizioni Orizzonte Medico (p. 151).

ANON., *USA, 18 June 1952—all surviving.*
The 26-year-old mother, from Weymouth, MA, had had three previous pregnancies, all normal and producing large infants weighing 8 to 9 lbs. (about 3630 to 4080g). From the second to the fourth month of her pregnancy she presented some minor problems. Because of her size at five months an X-ray was taken which revealed quads. She was admitted to hospital the following month. On July 17th she had mild contractions which subsequently stopped; they resumed the next day and became stronger. The babies, a girl followed by three boys, were born late in the evening at intervals of approximately one hour, 13 minutes and five minutes. Birthweights ranged from 1500 to 1800g. The afterbirth comprised two placental masses, each composed of two fused placental discs. Careful analysis of these membranes showed them to be different. One, that of the first- and third-born infants, was a fusion of two separate conceptions with two separate chorionic sacs. The second and fourth babies were intimately joined with placental vessels coursing

from one to the other, and there were amniotic membranes without chorions between the two gestation sacs. The evidence warrants the conclusion that these two boys were the result of MZ twinning and therefore that this was a TZ set. Note sequence of birth was girl, one of the MZ twin boys, boy, and then the second MZ twin. The babies were in good condition at birth and were making good progress at discharge.

Ryan, R.R., Wislocki, G.B. (1954) 'The birth of quadruplets, with an account of the placentas and fetal membranes.' *New England Journal of Medicine*, **250**, 755–758.

ANON., *USA, 6 January 1953—all surviving at 11 years.*
The mother was 32 years of age (previous pregnancies not reported). The prenatal course was uneventful except for the excessive enlargement of the abdomen, out of proportion to gestational age, which led to the suspicion of multiparity. This was confirmed by the location of several 'small parts' and different rates of fetal heartbeat. X-ray examination at seven months revealed four fetuses. Labour began spontaneously six weeks preterm and the mother was admitted to Bushwick Hospital, Brooklyn, NY. Four hours later the first three infants arrived at five minute intervals, followed in another 10 minutes by the fourth. There were three girls and a boy, weighing from 1445 to 1915g. The first baby born, who was also the heaviest, had a cleft palate. The first placenta was single with two cords and two amniotic sacs. The subsequent placentae were separate, each with its own cord. It was concluded that the quads were a TZ set. The cord bloods were tested but all were group A, type M, Rh+. The original report was read before the Medical Circle, New York, NY on 4 March 1955. It was subsequently published in October 1964, at which time the quads were described as being alive and well.

Ehrenpreis, B., Calcagno, J., Viviano, J., Berlin, H.S., DiNoie, J. (1964) 'Multiple pregnancy—surviving quadruplets.' *Medical Times*, **92**, 1053–1056.

JOUPPILA, *Finland, reported 1954—all surviving at 2 years.*
Miettinen (1954), in a review of triplet and quadruplet births in Finland from 1881 to 1952, listed the Jouppila children as the only quad set (out of a total of 37 liveborn cases) to survive past the age of 1 year. They were three boys and a girl (see photo overleaf), and their birthweights were in the 2000–2500g range. No placental analysis was undertaken, but from blood groupings and comparison of their physical characteristics it was judged that they were probably a TZ set.

Miettinen, M. (1954) 'On triplets and quadruplets in Finland.' *Acta Paediatrica*, **43** (Suppl. 99), 60–61; 76–77.

ANON., *Poland, 25 October 1954—all surviving at 20 years.*
These quads, born in Wroclaw, Poland are unique as the only MZ male set ever reported. Although their progress reports did not reach the literature in English until the 1970s, it is to the credit of the various scientists in several institutions in

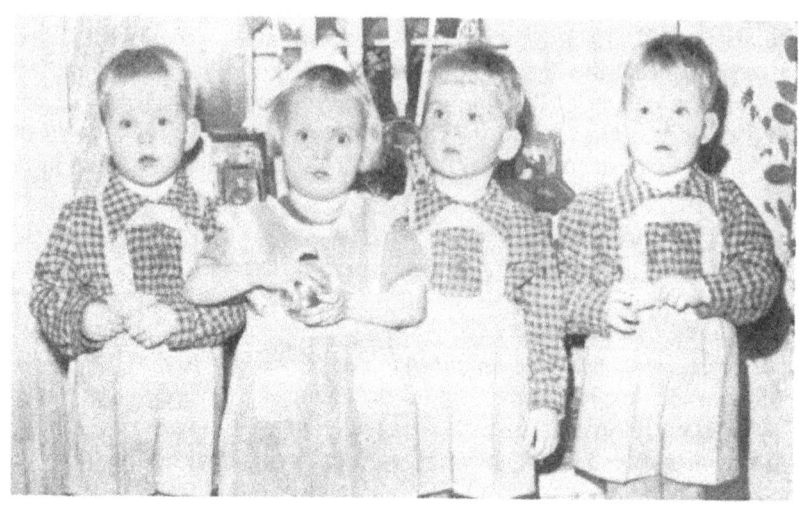

The **Jouppila** quads, age 2 years (Miettinen 1954)

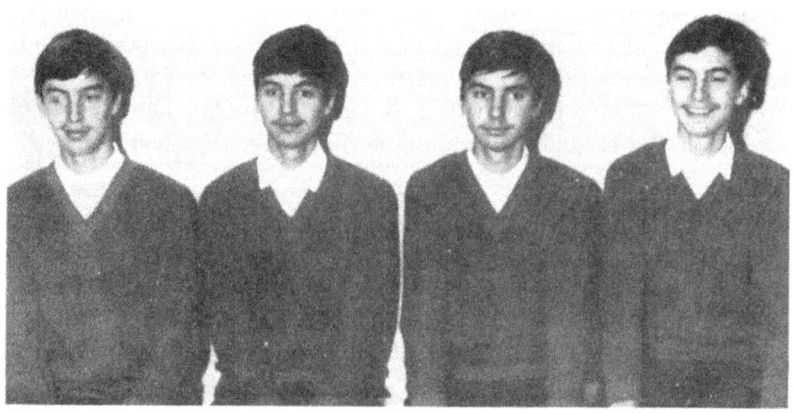

The 'Wroclaw quads' (Nowakowski 1974)

Poland that there is a better developmental record on these quads than on any other set with the possible exception of the Morloks. Despite the fact that one of the boys was injured during labour and suffered from one-sided paresis and deafness, living apart from the family for several years in special conditions, all the boys were reported to be similar in physical development (see Chapter 5, p. 49).

Glinkowa, K., Stachyra, J. (1970) 'Rozwoj fizyczny i umyslowy dzieci z ciazy czworaczej.' *Pediatria Polska*, **45**, 1121–1124.
Nowalowski, T.K. (1974) 'Uniovular quadruplets of Wroclaw.' *Acta Geneticae Medicae et Gemellologiae*, **22** (Suppl.), 154–158.

ANON., *Australia, 12 July 1956—no survival details.*
These quads were born in Bundaberg, Queensland. The mother was 32 years old and this was her first pregnancy. On April 5th 'the uterus was the size of a twenty-six weeks pregnancy, and as no fetal parts could be felt and as the period of amenorrhoea was approximately twenty-one weeks, the possibility of a multiple pregnancy was entertained'; X-ray examination revealed quads. She entered hospital at 36 weeks. Weak contractions were felt in the fortnight before the birth. After nine hours of labour a boy of 2580g was delivered. A second boy (2425g) followed an hour later, then a girl (1530g) another hour after that, and in a further 15 minutes another girl (2125g). 'Open ether' anaesthesia was used throughout. The condition of the second girl was poor but she improved rapidly. The afterbirth consisted of three placentae. The largest presented as a single mass but microscopic analysis of the common membrane between the two parts showed it to be composed of an amniotic layer on each surface with two chorionic layers between them. The four amniotic sacs were of approximately the same size and there was no communication between them.

Schmidt, E.E., Vickers, T.H. (1956) 'A case of multiple pregnancy: quadruplets.' *Medical Journal of Australia*, **1**, 791–794.

ANON., *England, 14 December 1957—all surviving.*
The mother, aged 37 and from Stepney, East London, had previously given birth to a boy and a set of DZ twins. At six months, because she was large for dates, an X-ray was taken. This showed three heads and four spines. The three heads could also be felt by palpation. She was admitted to hospital. A month later a second X-ray confirmed the presence of quads, and an electrocardiograph showed three separate tracings (the cardiologist gave assurance that this did not mean that the fourth baby was not alive). In the eighth month, although the mother showed no signs of labour there was gross overstretching of the uterus; the first baby was also a transverse lie and so it was decided to perform a caesarian section. There were two girls and two boys, and the birthweights ranged from 1760 to 2465g. The four babies were delivered in less than two minutes and 'each was carefully identified against the placental stump of its umbilical cord and given a symbol for later recognition'. Samples of cord blood were taken and similarly labelled. From detailed blood grouping and careful analysis of the placenta it was judged that the quads were a QZ set. They were named David, Thelma, Anthony and Beverley (see photo overleaf). Their progress in hospital was satisfactory and they were discharged on 26 January.

Hamilton, W.J., Brown, D., Spiers, B.G. (1959) 'Another case of quadruplets.' *Journal of Obstetrics and Gynaecology of the British Empire*, **66**, 409–412.

HOUROVA, *Czechoslovakia, 1 October 1959—all surviving.*
In an article on quintuplets, Tomas (1963) mentions this set as being the only quads to be born in Czechoslovakia between 1945 and 1959. They lived in Zbraslavice,

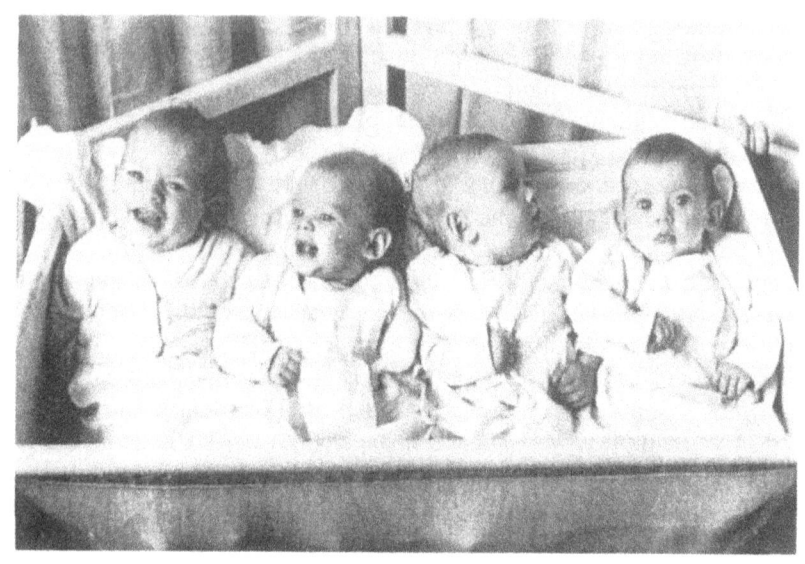

Quads reported by Hamilton *et al.* (1959), photographed at age 5 months
(*l–r*, David, Thelma, Anthony, Beverley)

near Kutna Hora in Bohemia. The two boys and two girls were cared for by the state, which supplied a nurse for them for three years. They had been well from birth and had developed normally.

Tomas, V. (1963) 'Les quintuplés aux pays Tchèques.' *Acta Geneticae Medicae et Gemellologiae*, **12**, 405–408.

ANON., *South Korea, 30 December 1959—all surviving at 5 years.*
This case, from the Il Sin Women's Hospital in Pusan, was reported in an Australian journal (Mackenzie 1965*). The mother was 31 years old and had had four previous pregnancies with successful deliveries. A midwife who examined her two days before the birth told her that she thought there were more than two babies. At first the mother refused to go into hospital but when labour commenced two days later she went to a private hospital. The babies, all girls and in good condition, were delivered by the midwife between 8.30 and 9.45pm. The mother's condition deteriorated in the next 24 hours, however, and her family allowed her to be transferred to the Women's Hospital where she died within two hours from eclampsia. The babies were also admitted but incubators were not available. Their weights at this time (birthweights were not given) ranged from 1596 to 2310g. Placental analysis indicated four separate amniotic sacs contained within a single chorion. Small cords led to small placental areas and presumably belonged to the two smaller babies. Microscopic sections of the membranes dividing the amniotic sacs were not made because of the delay before the placenta was received by the

Women's Hospital, but it was concluded that the quads were an MZ set. Their blood types were all group O, Rh+. They were the fourth female MZ set to be reported, and the first surviving quadruplets in Korea.

With careful nursing the babies progressed well but the father could not be pursuaded to take them home. Multiple births were not welcomed in his culture and quads were considered to be abnormal freaks. The father held the babies responsible for his wife's death and refused even to see them. His chances of finding a woman willing to marry him and undertake the care of seven children, four of them babies, would be slim. The quads were finally discharged to the care of an orphanage. Just before their second birthday they were adopted into an American family living in Minnesota. Their adoptive mother wrote before their fifth birthday that they were in good health, mentally alert and only the parents could tell them apart.

*Mackenzie's figures for Korea suggest that rates of multiple births are higher in that country than those reported for other Oriental groups.

Mackenzie, H.P. (1965) 'Surviving Korean quadruplets.' *Australia and New Zealand Journal of Obstetrics and Gynaecology*, **5**, 60–65.

ANON., *New Zealand, 31 March 1961—all surviving.*
At six months, due to an increasing disparity between gestation time and the size of the mother's uterus, X-ray examination was conducted and quads were diagnosed. The mother was admitted to hospital in Wellington on 24th March, at six-and-a-half months, and labour commenced a week later. The time interval between the rupturing of the first membranes and the birth of the last baby was just under an hour and a quarter. The babies were all girls and their weights ranged from 1760 to 2295g. Blood groupings showed three different patterns.

Quad	Blood grouping
1. Ann	A C− c+ D+ E+ M+ N− P+
2. Jill	A C+ c+ D+ E+ M+ N− P−
3. Helen	A C+ c+ D+ E+ M+ N+ P−
4. Colleen	A C+ c+ D+ E+ M+ N− P−

Although they had the same blood groupings, quads 2 and 4 were attached to different placentae and it is probable that this was a QZ set. The mother remained in hospital for a month and the progress of the babies was satisfactory.

Duncan, G.R., Kelly, J. (1961) 'Quadruplet pregnancy. A case report.' *New Zealand Medical Journal*, **60**, 375–376.

ANON., *France, 26 June 1961—all surviving.*
The mother was 38 years old and this was her third pregnancy. From the size of the uterus at six months a multiple gestation was suspected but this was not confirmed clinically until an X-ray taken at eight months revealed four fetuses. The mother was confined to bed in the last weeks of the pregnancy. Labour began

spontaneously but with weak contractions, and lasted 30 hours. The babies, three boys and a girl, were born 10 to 15 minutes apart. Birthweights ranged from 1640 to 2040g. Examination of the birth membranes suggested four chorionic and four amniotic sacs. Laboratory analysis confirmed that there was no communication between the vascular systems of the four placentae. One of the boys had blood type O, Rh+ while the other three infants were all type O, Rh−, a result which was confirmed several times. The children progressed well, leaving hospital at 3 months, and at 4 months were reported to be in good condition.

Toulouse, R., Toussaint, Cl., Le Clech, R., Grenier, A.J. (1961) 'Grossesse quadrigémellaire.' *Bulletin de la Fédération des Sociétés de Gynécologie et d'Obstétrique de Langue Française*, **13**, 663–666.

MEACHAM, *England, 3 January 1962—all surviving to adulthood.*
This set comprised two male and two female children. Their birthweights, in order of delivery, were as follows: Yana, 1590g; Lucille, 1590g; Edward, 1975g; Christopher, 1120g (data courtesy Guinness Books, from the *Southend Standard* newspaper). An article in *You* magazine (8 July 1984) reported on the quads, all still alive at 22 years.

BECKER, *Canada, 3 August 1962—all surviving.*
These quads, mentioned in the report on the McPherson quads (8 July 1972) in the *Daily Express* (10 July 1972), were born in Vancouver, BC. The birthweights and birth order (data courtesy Guinness Books) were 2465g (girl), 2265g (boy), 2240g (boy), 2015g (girl).

GENAIN, *reported 1963—all surviving to adulthood.*
The mother was 31 years old and had no other children. By the fifth month her doctor diagnosed twins, but she felt that she would have three or four. The babies, all girls, were born in hospital within 17 minutes of one another; by her dates they were about a month preterm. The birthweights were approximately 2040, 1505, 1930 and 1360g. The mother wanted to look after her four babies and bring them up; however, the father was shocked by their arrival. The mother had almost complete responsibility for them when they went home at 5 weeks, with a little home and neighbourly help. She kept records on their progress from 6 months. They were toilet trained for the daytime by 20 months, but had nocturnal enuresis until the ages of 16 or 18 years.

Results of intelligence tests at 10 years and details of elementary and high school progress were reported by Bayley (1963) (see Chapter 5, pp. 56–57 and Table 5.VII, p. 59). As young women they all developed schizophrenia, and they were made the subjects of a longitudinal study examining their behavioural, psychiatric, neurological and biochemical development. Particular interest centred on the fact that they were monozygotic, discordant for the severity of their disorders, and functioning as well as they ever had since the onset of the disorder. Mirsky and Duncan-Johnson (1984) proposed the hypothesis, from these and other case studies, that given a schizophrenic diathesis, life events can modify (reduce or enhance) the severity of the phenotypic expression of the disorder.

Bayley, N. (1963) 'Intellectual and physical development.' *In:* Rosenthal, D. (Ed.) *The Genain Quadruplets.* New York: Basic Books.
Buchsbaum, M.S., Mirsky, A.F., DeLisi, L.E., Morihisa, J., Karson, C.N., Mendelson, W.B., King, A.C., Johnson, J., Kessler, R. (1984) 'The Genain quadruplets: electrophysiological, positron emission, and X-ray tomographic studies.' *Psychiatry Research*, **13**, 95–108.
DeLisi, L.E., Mirsky, A.F., Buchsbaum, M.S., van Kammen, D.P., Berman, K.F., Caton, C., Kafka, M.S., Ninan, P.T., Phelps, B.H., Karoum, F., Ko, G.N., Korpi, E.R., Linnoila, M., Sheinan, M., Wyatt, R.J. (1984) 'The Genain quadruplets 25 years later: a diagnostic and biochemical followup.' *Psychiatry Research*, **13**, 59–76.
Mirsky, A.F., Duncan-Johnson, C.C. (1984) 'Nature versus nurture in schizophrenia: the struggle continues.' *Integrative Psychiatry*, **2**, 137–141.
—— DeLisi, L.E., Buchsbaum, M.S., Quinn, O.W., Schwerdt, P., Siever, L.J., Mann, L., Weingartner, H., Zec, R., Sostek, A., Alterman, I., Revere, V., Dawson, S.D., Zahn, T.P. (1984) 'The Genain quadruplets: psychological studies.' *Psychiatry Research*, **13**, 77–93.
Rosenthal, D. (Ed.) (1963) *The Genain Quadruplets.* New York: Basic Books.

ANON., *USA, 3 June 1964—none surviving beyond 2 days.*
The mother (Mrs M.P.) lived in Brooklyn, NY, was 30 years old and had two children already. X-ray at six months suggested a triplet pregnancy, a diagnosis which was not revised until the actual birth. Labour began in the seventh month and the mother was admitted to hospital. It was nine hours from the onset of labour to the birth of the first baby, a male of 1275g. A girl weighing only 905g was delivered 15 minutes later and another girl, of 1135g, three minutes after that. The fourth baby, again a female, was discovered and delivered five minutes later (birthweight not given). There were four amniotic sacs but only two chorions, indicating a DZ origin. All four infants showed respiratory distress and despite intensive care all died within two days. The case was reported 'in order to encourage the keeping of similar records for eventual definitive statistical and aetiological studies which might throw more light on a neglected subject.'

Giorlando, S.W., Hall, J.E. (1966) 'Biovular quadruplets.' *International Surgery*, **46**, 292–294.

O'CONNELL, *Ireland, 23 January 1965—all alive at 9 days.*
The *Irish Times* (1 February 1965) reported the birth of quads (two male, two female) at Limerick Regional Maternity Hospital. Their weights at birth were not given, but at 9 days they were as follows: Catherine (990g), Gerard (1530g), John (1675g), Margaret (1360g). The mother was aged 36 years.

ANON., *Scotland, 15 May 1965—all surviving at 9 months.*
The mother, who lived in Aberdeen, was aged 29 years and already had two sets of twin girls, all alive and well having been delivered at 40 and 38 weeks respectively. This third pregnancy was planned and she had taken out insurance cover. Multiparity was suspected at 18 weeks; this was confirmed by X-ray which revealed quadruplets. She was admitted to hospital and remained there until the birth, which

occurred at 33 weeks by her menstrual history. Labour was spontaneous and the infants, three girls and a boy, were delivered by caesarian section within two minutes. Birthweights ranged from 1635 to 1870g. From blood sample analysis it was thought that this was a TZ set. Condition of the babies at birth was reasonable, although the last born had considerable respiratory distress. They were discharged at 66 days. At 9 months the children were all in excellent health and their psychomotor development was within normal limits.

Fullerton, W.T., Hytten, F.E., Klopper, A.I., McKay, E. (1965) 'A case of quadruplet pregnancy.' *Journal of Obstetrics and Gynaecology of the British Commonwealth*, **72**, 791–796.

ANON., *New Zealand, 20 December 1965—all surviving.*
Details of this set were provided by Prof D.G. Bonham of the National Women's Hospital, Auckland *(personal communication)*. The mother was 29 years old and had two adopted children. She became pregnant following HPG (human pituitary growth hormone) therapy for infertility, and at 30 weeks was admitted to the National Women's Hospital after a threatened abortion. The babies were delivered a week later at 222 days. The first born was a boy of 1300g, followed by two girls, both 1530g, and last another boy of 1250g. They were diagnosed to be a QZ set.

ANON., *USA, 1965 (undated)—all surviving.*
The mother conceived after treatment with gonadotropins, and following a successful pregnancy she gave birth to three girls and a boy. Birthweights were from 1240 to 1800g. There were four amnions and four chorions, indicating that they were a QZ set. Mother and children progressed well.

Neuwirth, R.S., Todd, W.D., Turksoy, R.N., Vandewiele, R.L. (1965) 'Successful quadruplet pregnancy in a patient treated with human menopausal gonadotropins.' *American Journal of Obstetrics and Gynecology*, **91**, 982–984.

ALEXANDER, *New Zealand, 2 September 1967—all surviving at 22 years.*
The mother was 37 years old and already had two sons aged 9 and 11. Her third pregnancy was ectopic. Multiparity was not suspected until 35 weeks. She was referred for radiography and the X-ray revealed quads. She was straight away admitted to the National Women's Hospital, Auckland. At 40 weeks there were still no signs of spontaneous labour and an examination was conducted to determine whether to induce labour or to perform a caesarian section. The latter course was decided on and the four infants were delivered safely. There was a large single placenta with four separate cord insertions and three amniotic sacs. The last two babies shared one of these—their cords showed marked entanglement with a true knot present. All four babies showed identical blood typing across eight separate groups, indicating that they were probably an MZ set. The birthweights were 1940, 1810, 1640 and 1760g, and all were in good condition. The Apgar scores were as follows.

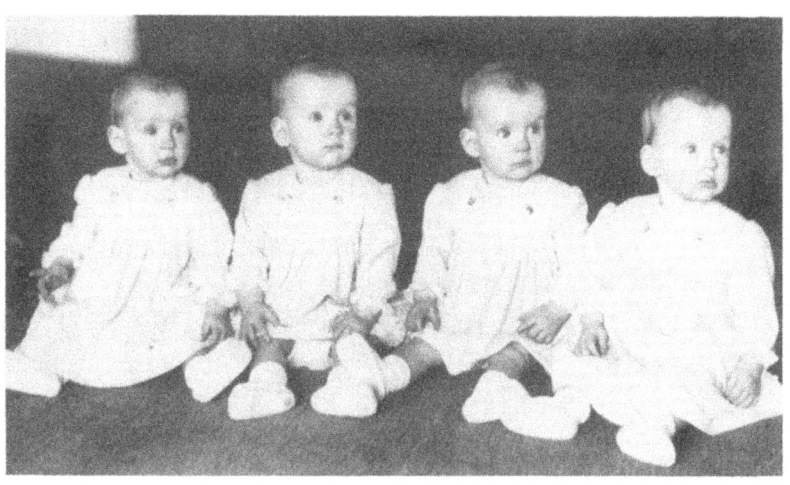

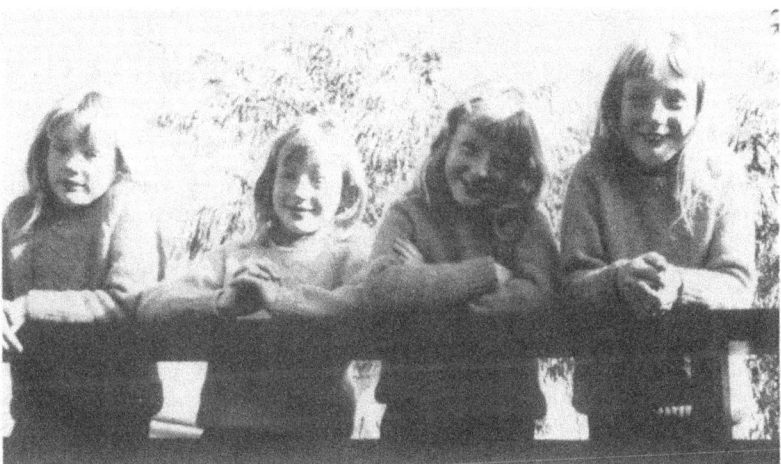

The **Alexander** quads: *above,* at about 1 year (*l–r,* Elizabeth, Delwyn, Kathryn, Louise); *below,* aged 8 years (*l–r,* Kathryn, Elizabeth, Louise, Delwyn). (Photos from the personal collection of Mrs Jean Alexander)

Apgar	Baby 1	Baby 2	Baby 3	Baby 4
1 minute	6	3–4	1–2	3
5 minutes	8	7	—	5
10 minutes	10	9–10	10	7

The mother's postoperative progress was uneventful and she was discharged fit and well after two weeks. The babies were kept in the hospital longer than usual while suitable accommodation for the family of eight was found. A paediatric check at 26 weeks indicated good progress. All four were reaching and grasping, bearing weight on their feet well, and almost sitting unaided.

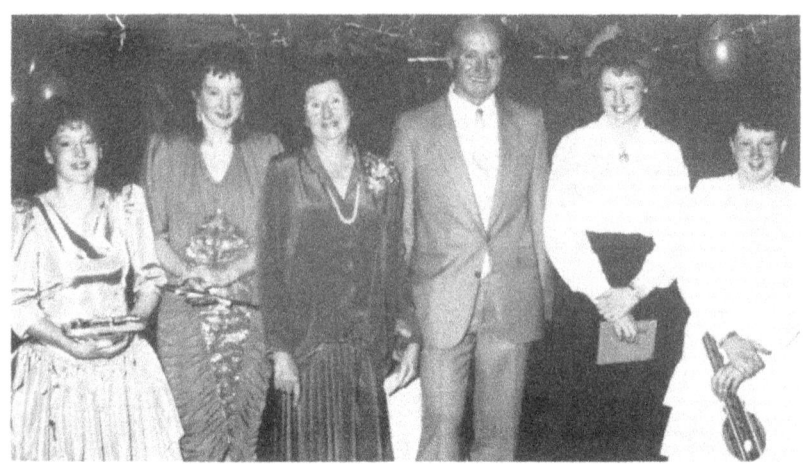

The **Alexander** quads photographed on their 21st birthday (*l–r*, Kathryn, Elizabeth, parents Jean and Ron Alexander, Louise, Delwyn). (Photo by Sirrom Studios, Browns Bay Photographers; from the personal collection of Mrs Jean Alexander)

Their subsequent progress was summarized in a recent article* in the *New Zealand Herald* (12 September 1989), which reported the mother's death, at 59 years, 'one week after her four daughters celebrated their 22nd birthday'.

Although the quads strained the family budget, wellwishing Aucklanders helped out. The quads were showered with gifts including baby clothing, a food company sent them a big load of baby provisions and a businessman donated two twin prams.

Despite all the publicity, their parents were determined to see the quads lead normal lives. They were educated at Westlake Girls' High School, and Mrs Alexander refused to let them be used in any advertising. "I didn't want them brought up any different from their brothers," she once said. Mrs Alexander made a conscious effort to share herself among her children and to raise them as individuals—"Otherwise they'd be just like little pets."

Elizabeth now works for an electronics company, Louise married a year ago, Kathryn is a trainee nurse and Delwyn is married with two children.

*Reproduced by kind permission of the *New Zealand Herald*, Auckland, NZ.

Fraser, F.A. (1968) *Case Records and Commentaries Presented for Membership of the Royal College of Obstetricians and Gynaecologists*, National Women's Hospital, Auckland, NZ.

ANON., *Switzerland, reported 1967—three surviving.*
The mother had had one normal pregnancy five years previously. She received hormone treatment (clomiphene) for two years before this birth. She was hospitalized briefly in early pregnancy. The presence of quads was shown by X-ray at 30 weeks. Labour was induced at 35 weeks but then it was decided to perform a caesarian section. The quads—three boys and one girl—had birthweights of 2200, 1550, 1800 and 1580g. One died at 12 days but the others were still alive at the time of the report.

Fankhauser, B. (1967) 'Bericht über Vierlingsgravidität nach Clomiphenbehandlung.' *Archiv für Gynäkologie*, **204**, 279–280.

Hochuli, E., Fankhauser, B. (1967) 'Vierlinggravidität und -geburt nach Clomiphenbehandlung. Ein kasuistischer Beitrag.' *Geburtshilfe und Frauenheilkunde*, **27**, 1043–1051.

ANON., *Nigeria, c.1967–1969—no survival details.*
One quadruplet delivery was reported along with a series of 44 sets of triplets in a study of higher multiple births in Ibadan, Nigeria. There were two placentae, each with a single chorion containing two amniotic sacs. Two boys were attached to one placenta and two girls to the other. Blood tests were not conducted and no further details were recorded.

Nylander, P.P.S., Corney, G. (1973) 'Placentation and zygosity of triplets and higher multiple births in Ibadan, Nigeria.' *Annals of Human Genetics*, **34**, 417–426.

ANON., *Austria, 1 March 1968—three surviving.*
Two boys and two girls were born by vaginal delivery at intervals of one hour 40 minutes, 15 minutes and three minutes. Birthweights were from 900 to 1470g. They were taken to a children's clinic for special nursing but one girl died at 3 days. Detailed blood analyses conducted at the World Health Organization's National Blood Group Reference Laboratory in Vienna showed that this was a QZ set, as both members of each same-sex pair had different blood groups.

Mayr, W.R., Pausch, V., Mickerts, D. (1969) 'Serologische Befunde an viereiigen Vierlingen.' *Wiener Klinische Wochenschrift*, **81**, 687–689.

ANON., *England, 19 April 1970—all surviving.*
A 28-year-old mother, whose first child had been born following clomiphene citrate treatment, was given pituitary gonadotropins two years later after further citrate treatment had proved unsuccessful. Following the second course of treatment, she complained of acute abdominal pain which was confined to the iliac fossae. Ovarian masses were palpable abdominally and a diagnosis of the 'hyperstimulation syndrome' was made. The symptom gradually settled and some days later the result of a serological pregnancy test was positive. At 25 weeks there was a gross discrepancy between the size of the uterus and the period of gestation. Triplets were suspected and a sonogram confirmed this impression, although only one longitudinal scan was made. Labour commenced at 32 weeks and the babies—three boys and a girl—were born by vaginal delivery at approximately 10 minute intervals. Birthweights 1445, 1530, 1615 and 1700g. There were three amniotic sacs.

Atlay, R.D., Pennington, G.W. (1971) 'The use of clomiphene citrate and pituitary gonadotropin in successive pregnancies: the Sheffield quadruplets.' *American Journal of Obstetrics and Gynecology*, **109**, 402–407.

ANON., *Israel, reported 1970—two sets: (i) non-viable; (ii) two surviving at 1 year.*
Hack *et al.* (1970) reported on one set of quads and one set of sextuplets conceived after fertility drug treatment at the Tel-Hashomer Government Hospital, Tel Aviv, and which were born immature at 154 and 157 days respectively. A second set of

quads carried to 198 days. Only two female babies lived. Their birthweights were 1190 and 1270g. At 6 and 12 months they were below the third percentile of normal development for height and weight.

Hack, M., Brish, M., Serr, D.M., Insler, V., Lunenfeld, B. (1970) 'Outcome of pregnancy after induced ovulation.' *Journal of the American Medical Association*, **211**, 791–797.

ANON., *USA, 19 May 1971—three surviving.*
The mother, who lived in Denver, CO, was 23 years old and had one other child. Multiple pregnancy was diagnosed at 27 weeks and she was hospitalized. Labour began spontaneously at 30 weeks and after a five hour first stage she gave birth to four babies in nine minutes without analgesia. The babies—all girls—were small, weighing from 735 to 1190g. The last born was the smallest and died at 48 hours of respiratory distress syndrome. The report of the birth membranes is confusing. The first two babies had 'a single sac' and the other two had 'separate sacs' (presumably amniotic sacs). Histological examination revealed a common chorion for three of the babies, with the fourth in a separate chorion. Thus, according to the report, the pregnancy was dichorionic and triamniotic, and therefore rather interesting. One baby had a separate chorion and amnion, while three babies shared a chorionic sac, two of these sharing one of the two amniotic sacs within that chorionic sac. The three surviving babies were discharged from hospital at 6 to 8 weeks.

McFee, J.G., Lord, E.L., Jeffrey, R.L., O'Meara, O.P., Josepher, H.J., Butterfield, J., Thompson, H.E. (1974) 'Multiple gestations of high fetal number.' *Obstetrics and Gynaecology*, **44**, 99–106.

McPHERSON, *England, 8 July 1972—all surviving.*
This set comprised three girls—Fiona (birthweight 2295g), Kirsten (2695g), Rachel (2125g)—and a boy—Guy (2550g). The *Daily Express* (10 July 1972), which published photos of the set, reported them as the heaviest on record at that time (see, however: Norriss, 28 March 1889; Anon., 27 July 1907). The mother, who was aged 28 years and already had a 4-year-old daughter, had been on a course of fertility drug treatment. She was quoted as saying:

"I made up my mind I would not have a premature birth and that the babies would not be underweight. As it turned out, I went to 37 weeks—one week over full pregnancy—and that is why they are so heavy and healthy."

The birth took place at Liverpool Maternity Hospital, and took only five minutes (though it was not stated whether delivery was vaginal or by caesarian section).

ANON., *USA, 7 December 1972—all surviving.*
The 28-year-old, Black mother from Denver, CO, commenced prenatal care at nine weeks. This was her seventh pregnancy after three live births and three abortions. Her uterus enlarged out of all proportion to dates; at 31 weeks it was described as term-sized and she began to complain of difficulty in locomotion. One week later an ultrasonic scan was interpreted as indicating a twin gestation. At

33 weeks she was admitted to hospital and an X-ray revealed four skeletons and ultrasound showed four heads. Labour began spontaneously at 35 weeks. The first baby was born after three hours, the other three in the next 20 minutes. There were three boys and a girl, weighing from 1340 to 2390g. There were four placentae, four chorions and four amnions. The babies did well and were discharged at 2 to 4 weeks.

McFee, J.G., Lord, E.L., Jeffrey, R.L., O'Meara, O.P., Josepher, H.J., Butterfield, J., Thompson, H.E. (1974) 'Multiple gestations of high fetal number.' *Obstetrics and Gynaecology*, **44**, 99–106.

ANON., *England, 19 May 1973—all surviving.*
The mother lived in Surrey (her age is not reported) and had had one normal pregnancy four years earlier. She had been treated with clomiphene and pergonal. At eight weeks her uterus was larger than expected and she was warned of the possibility of a multiple pregnancy. Ultrasonic scanning in the third month revealed three fetuses and two repeat scans at monthly intervals did not change this diagnosis. The mother was admitted to hospital at 28 weeks. Labour began spontaneously at 35 weeks and two hours later the first baby was delivered, a boy of 1985g, followed by another boy of 1930g, then a girl of 1955g and finally a third boy of 1845g. In all the births took 20 minutes. The report states that the mother . .

. . was relieved that there were only four babies and not five and was very pleased they were all alive and appeared healthy. She rang her husband herself to tell him about her wonderful experience of giving birth to live quadruplets after only a three-hour labour. Yet, at the third day when she was taken to visit the babies in the Special Care Unit she found it hard to realise that she had four vigorous healthy babies.

The parents and their small daughter planned to have a short holiday together before preparing to welcome home the large addition to their family. The babies were discharged at about 1 month of age, in pairs and three days apart so that the mother could get used to coping with the extra work and her daughter could accept the babies being home. The mother visited the hospital three times following her discharge and apparently was coping well with the aid of a home help.

Jackson, J. (1976) 'Case study: quadruplets.' *Midwives Chronicle and Nursing Notes*, (May), 1060.

ANON., *USA, reported 1974—all surviving.*
The mother was 27 years old and lived in New York. Four years previously, following fertility drug treatment, she had given birth to a healthy baby girl. She subsequently sought further treatment for a second pregnancy. Ultrasonogram at 18 weeks confirmed the presence of quads. She remained on bed-rest at home until 28 weeks when she was admitted to hospital at the Cornell University Medical College. She was acquainted with the Lamaze method of childbirth and wanted to stay awake during the births. This was possible as no complications occurred. The delivery went smoothly and no anaesthesia was required. The babies—one boy and three girls, weighing from 1760 to 1960g—were born at 34 weeks, an hour after the

onset of labour, by spontaneous vaginal delivery. There were four separate placentae, indicating that this was a QZ set. The mother breast-fed all the babies, and they were discharged from hospital at 3 weeks.

Lauerson, N.H., Buchman, M., Beling, C.G. (1974) 'Successful quadruplet pregnancy following ovulation induced with human menopausal gonadotropin and human chorionic gonadotropin.' *Acta Obstetrica et Gynecologica Scandinavica*, **53**, 387–391.

KYRIAZIS, *Australia, 9 April 1974—all surviving.*
The parents were immigrants from Egypt who had been living in South Australia for four years. The mother was 28 years old and had three other children. She had been hospitalized for 11 weeks. A birth team of more than 12 specialists was formed and they were on call for over six weeks until the birth, which was to be by caesarian section at a pre-arranged time. The first to be delivered was a girl of 2430g, followed by three boys, the lightest of whom weighed 2010g. The birth was monitored by closed-circuit television, watched by staff, medical students, and a woman journalist from the *Australian Women's Weekly* (her report being published in the edition of 24 April 1974).

ANON., *USSR, 20 May 1974—all surviving at 2½ years.*
The mother, aged 36, had two sons from two previous pregnancies. The quads, four girls named Vala, Lena, Victoria and Lisa, were born at the Children's (Maternity) Hospital in Zaporozh'ye in the Ukraine. No details of the prenatal or birth history were given. Birthweights were 1250, 1050, 1300 and 920g. Analysis suggested that this was a QZ set. Neonatal care for the first 30 days was reported in detail. At 2 months 6 days the quads were discharged from hospital and then came under the supervision of the Children's Polyclinic. All branches of the medical services contributed to their care and development. A nurse and nurse aid provided all-round care in the first year and a paediatrician visited the children at least once a week. Community support came from the milk bank and help was provided at home without charge.

All the infants had several medical anomalies and illnesses in their first year. All had recurrent anaemia which responded to treatment, all had dysplasia of the joints of the pelvis, all had umbilical hernia, three had recurrent respiratory illness, three had rickets and two had flat feet. Despite these physical illnesses, neurological status was without pathology and psychomotor development was normal in three quads but in the other (Lisa) it was somewhat delayed. Those three spoke their first words at 8, 9 and 10 months but Lisa was slower to talk. At 2½ years Vala spoke better than her sisters and was the 'leader' of the group. Her physical development was no more than 0.5 SD below the mean for that age; Victoria and Lena were respectively 1.0 SD and 1.5–2.0 SD below the mean; while Lisa was 2.5 SD below the mean and very small for her age.

Shcherbak, I.G., Neishtadt, A.E., Shpiller, E.E., Mel'nikoya, A.S., Zelenskiy, V.M. (1978) 'Certain results of observations of the development of quadruplets.' *Pediatriya*, **1**, 73–75.

STRUVE, *USA, 12 June 1974—all surviving at 7 years.*
On 5 June 1982, the (American) *Guinness Book of World Records* brought together 16 quads (*i.e.* four sets) and 147 triplets on 'a quiet side street in North Hollywood' (*Los Angeles Times*, 7 June 1982) to establish the record for the largest number of such multiples ever assembled at one time (see overleaf). The Struve quads—Kevin, Kristina, Todd and Tonya—were among the participants in this event, which took place one week before their eighth birthday. (Unfortunately, no details other than the names and birthdate are available for any of the four sets. Information and press cutting courtesy Guinness Books.)

ANON., *France, 20 September 1974—all surviving.*
The mother was 33 years old and this was her first pregnancy. Multiple pregnancy was confirmed by ultrasonograph which showed three heads; the fourth was detected by X-ray shortly before the birth. The babies were delivered by caesarian section at 36 weeks. The birthweights varied quite markedly: 2040, 1400, 1930 and 1210g. All four were boys (Jacques, Mickaël, Stève, Stéphen). The placenta was reported to have a single chorion and four amniotic sacs. This evidence of MZ status was supported by serological analysis which showed that the babies all had the same blood groups across 10 components. The mother had been given a sodium-deficient diet for the latter part of her pregnancy and the report deals with the problems of such a restriction.

Lelong-Tissier, M.C., Retbi, J.M., Dehan, M., Vial, M., Frydman, R., Gagilan, J.C. (1977) 'Hyponatrémie maternofoetale carentielle par régime désodé.' *Archives Françaises de Pédiatrie*, **34**, 64–70.

TANNER, *England, ?May 1975—all alive at 2 weeks.*
These four girls—believed to comprise two pairs of MZ 'twins'—were born at the Poole General Hospital, Dorset. A local newspaper, the *Bournemouth Echo* (press cutting, full date not recorded, courtesy Guinness Books), published a photograph of the quads being tended in the special care baby unit, reporting that they were 'progressing well . . . and regaining their initial, though quite natural, weight loss'.

BERGQUIST, *USA, 7 September 1975—all surviving.*
These quads were born by vaginal delivery at the University of Minnesota Hospitals, Minneapolis, MN. They were the result of spontaneous ovulation. All four were girls, and in order of delivery their respective birthweights were: Ann (2290g), Elizabeth (2430g), Mary (2430g), Rebecca (2610g)—a total of 9760g. Prior to the birth of the Takeda quads (2 October 1978), they were quoted by the *Guinness Book of Records* as the heaviest set on record (see, however, Norriss, 28 March 1889; Anon., 27 July 1907). The parents already had one 2-year-old daughter. (Information courtesy Guinness Books.)

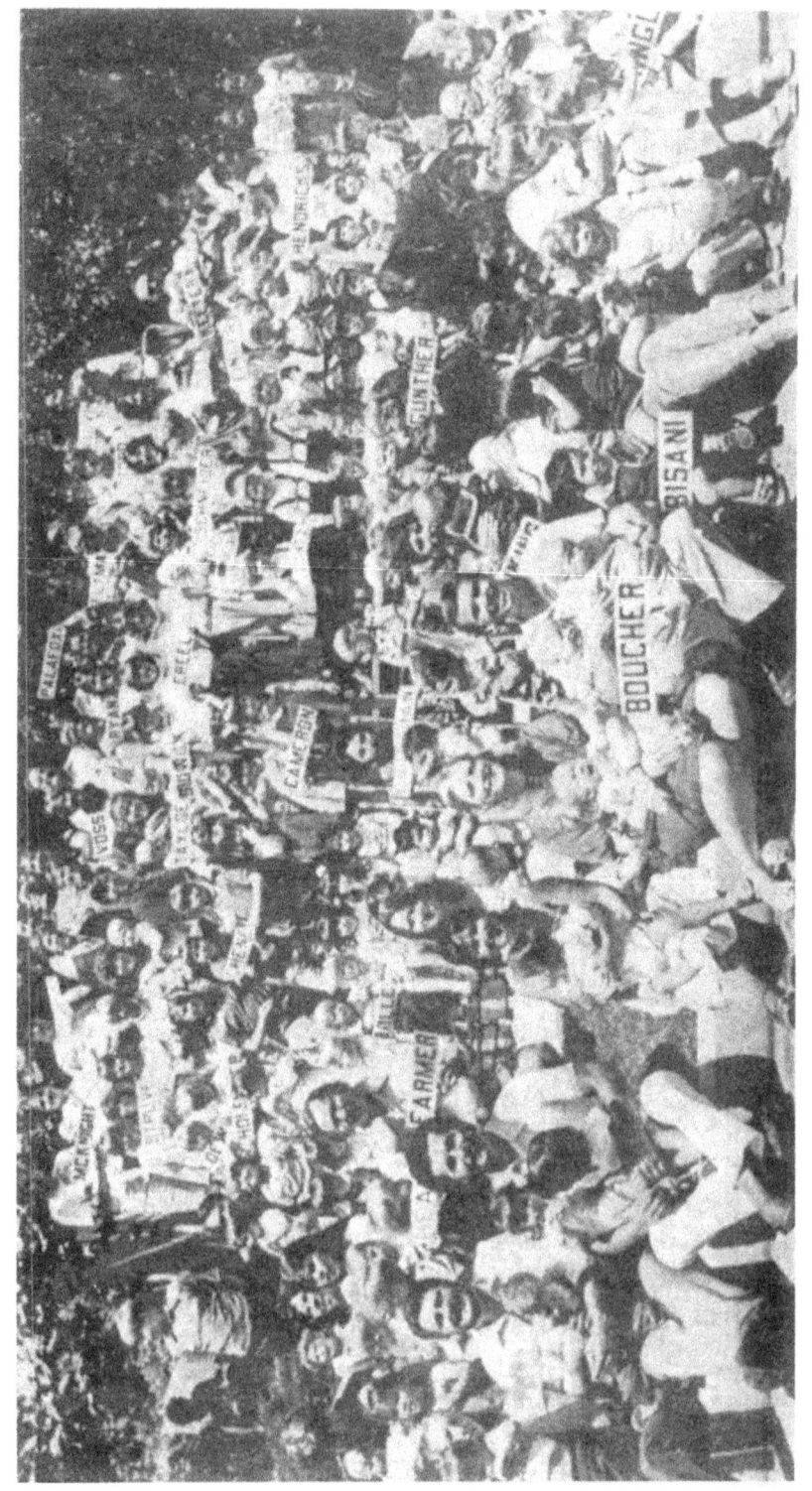

Part of the gathering of triplets and quads brought together in North Hollywood, CA, on 5 June 1982 by the *Guinness Book of World Records*. The **Struve** quads (12 June 1974) and the **Holsather** quads (24 February 1977) can be seen toward the top left-hand corner of this photograph, which appeared in the *Los Angeles Times* of 7 June 1982 (photo: Martha Traeger)

ANON., *Israel, reported 1976—three sets: (i) all aborted; (ii) only one surviving; (iii) all surviving.*
Reporting on all women treated for infertility in the Assaf Harofe Government Hospital, Zerifin, Israel between 1968 and 1975 (a total of 143 pregnancies in 110 women), Caspi *et al.* (1976) referred to three quadruplet gestations in the 112 pregnancies which lasted more than 20 weeks. (The number of fetuses in early miscarriages was not stated.) Because this was a summary of all births the quadruplet data were not detailed but they can be extracted in part from the tables.
1. One set was born at 22 weeks, each weighing about 300g. They all died and their sex was not recorded.
2. The second set was born at 29 weeks. They were all boys and the birthweights, read from a graph, appear to range from 1100 to 1190g. Only the first-born survived.
3. The third set—three girls and one boy—were born at 38 weeks. The birthweights were approximately 1980 to 2400g. From the general statements in the report it can be concluded that they were a QZ set and that they were all normal, healthy babies.

Caspi, E., Ronen, J., Schreyer, P., Goldberg, M.D. (1976) 'The outcome of pregnancy after gonadotropin therapy.' *British Journal of Obstetrics and Gynaecology*, **83**, 967–973.

KUHN, *USA, 3 January 1976—three surviving.*
These quads were born at St Mary Hospital, Quincy, IL, by spontaneous vaginal delivery, within the space of only nine minutes. Confirmation of this was obtained from the hospital. All four were boys (Curtis, Craig, Christopher, Colin); according to the mother, the three who survived were MZ 'triplets'. (Information courtesy Guinness Books.)

ANON., *England, 1976—two cases: (i) one surviving; (ii) three surviving.*
This report came from the Department of Paediatrics at the John Radcliffe Hospital, Oxford. The two mothers had concurrent pregnancies, the dates of conception differing by only two weeks. In both cases ovulation had been induced by treatment with human chorionic gonadotrophin (HCG), and in both cases episodes of preterm labour occurred at 28 weeks and were stopped by administration of salbutamol.

Case 1. The mother had a history of anorexia nervosa and anovulatory infertility. In the two weeks following the first episode of labour fulminating toxaemia developed, and at 30 weeks, due to rising blood pressure, retinal artery spasm, rising blood urea and increasing proteinuria, it was decided to perform a caesarian section. Time from induction of anaesthesia to the delivery of the last baby was seven minutes. The birthweights were 1205, 1035, 720 and 820g respectively. The first-born developed mild respiratory distress but recovered well. The other three, however, all developed severe hyaline membrane disease and bilateral pneumothoraces, dying at 48 hours, 14 days and 28 days respectively.

Case 2. This was the mother's second pregnancy; the first had also followed HCG treatment and resulted in a normal singleton birth. At 34 weeks she had an antepartum haemorrhage which tests showed to be of fetal origin, and an emergency caesarian section was performed. The first-born infant was white and profoundly asphyxiated as a result of the haemorrhage; it lived only 8 hours. The other three had no further problems and were said to be developing normally. The birthweights ranged from 1620 to 1850g.

The report, by Salisbury and colleagues, focused primarily on the procedures adopted in advance of the birth. It was planned to have four teams at each delivery, one for each infant, comprising two paediatricians and an experienced nurse. In addition, a biochemistry technician would be on standby to take and analyse cord-blood samples. To ensure the attendance of such a large number of staff at short notice an availability list was maintained on the special care baby unit from the 25th week of gestation onwards. In the light of their experiences with these two cases the authors concluded:

An intensive care neonatal unit in a busy maternity hospital must have a degree of flexibility that can adapt to an unpredictable workload. However, multiple pre-term births at any time impose great strain on both staff and equipment, and it was the concurrence of 2 sets of quads which led us to make the special arrangements outlined in this report. Despite these arrangements only 4 of the 8 infants survived.

It may be that borderline viability [multiple] births are at an unavoidable disadvantage compared with singleton births. However, if a pre-term low birthweight infant from a multiple pregnancy is individually to have a chance of intact survival similar to a singleton low birthweight infant he will need the same intensity of medical and nursing care from the moment of delivery through the early neonatal period. Most units will be able to provide intensive care for twin pre-term infants. However, for higher multiple births additional equipment and personnel are required. Efforts should therefore be made for women with multiple pregnancies to be delivered in regional centres where adequate staff and neonatal equipment are available.

While it is impossible to show that our expenses and efforts modified the outcome for these quadruplets, the additional nursing, medical and technical staff were able to concentrate on the care of these babies without compromising the routine care provided for the other babies in the Special Care Baby Unit.

Salisbury, D.M., Jones, R.W.A., Townshend, P., Baum, J.D. (1977) 'Paediatric preparation for multiple premature births.' *Early Human Development*, **1**, 39–45.

ANON., *Denmark, 19 August 1976—no survival data.*
The mother, who lived in Copenhagen, had been receiving menotropinum (Humegon) and choriongonadotropinum (Physex) treatment for secondary amenorrhoea. The case report states that . .

The last injections were given in the first week of December and on the 2nd and the 10th of January. The first day of the last menstrual period was the 14th of December. The patient had intercourse with her husband in the days 22nd–26th of December and again on the 14th of January and not in between as he was away from home in this period.

In mid-February a pregnancy test proved positive. X-ray examination at the beginning of August confirmed the diagnosis of a multiple gestation. Two weeks later (at about the 36th week) spontaneous labour commenced and a caesarian section was carried out. The babies—two girls and two boys—were in good condition and according to sex and blood group analysis were quadrizygotic. The birthweights ranged from 1420 to 1770g. Measurements of the infants and tests of cord-serum α-fetoprotein (AFP) levels led the authors to the conclusion that . .

. . judged from the anamnestic data of stimulation with Humegon and Physex, the clinical observations and the AFP concentration, infant D has a 2–3 weeks lower gestational age than A, B and C. Infant D may therefore be an example of superfetatio. We thus believe that the first conception occurred after a spontaneous ovulation about the 26th of December and that the second conception occurred after a medically induced ovulation about the 14th of January.

Nørgaard-Pedersen, B., Møller, J., Trolle, D., Sørensen, S.A. (1976) 'α-Fetoprotein concentration in cord blood from twins and from a set of quadruplets—a case of superfetatio?' *Human Heredity*, **26**, 72–78.

ANON., *USA, reported 1977—all surviving.*
The mother was referred at 32 weeks to a hospital in Charleston, SC, with a diagnosis of twins. Ultrasound showed three fetal heads while an X-ray revealed quads. A team of doctors and nurses was assembled and it was decided to carry out a caesarian section after the commencement of labour. The operation was eventually performed after two weeks of intermittent contractions, and the infants were delivered at one minute intervals. The first two were males with weights of 1940 and 2050g, and the second pair were females of 1227 and 1700g. The gestational age was 34 weeks. The placenta of Infant 1 was attached to that of Infant 4 and the placenta of Infant 3 was attached to that of Infant 3. Section of the membranes between the two placental masses showed that they were diamniotic and dichorionic. Infant 3 had hyaline membrane disease but recovered well and all infants were progressing well on discharge.

Purohit, D.M., Levkoff, A.H., Pai, S. (1977) 'Management of multifetal gestation.' *Pediatric Clinics of North America*, **24**, 481–490.

HOLSATHER, *USA, 24 February 1977—all surviving at 5 years.*
The Holsather quads (Elizabeth, Rachel, Rebecca, Joseph) were the second set of quads represented in the *Guinness Book of World Records* gathering on 5 June 1982 (see Struve, 12 June 1974; and photograph, p. 156).

ANON., *USA, reported 1978—all surviving.*
The mother was 30 years old with one previous child and had been treated with clomiphene citrate five months before this pregnancy. At 35 weeks an ultrasonogram showed four fetuses and a large single anterior low placenta, and the mother was admitted to hospital. Elective caesarian section with epidural analgesia was carried out at 38 weeks. The babies—three girls and a boy, weighing from 1400 to 2500g—were delivered at three-minute intervals and crying was immediate.

Craft, J.B., Levinson, G., Shnider, S.M. (1978) 'Anaesthetic considerations in caesarian section for quadruplets.' *Canadian Anaesthetists Society Journal*, **25**, 236–239.

ANON., *Japan, 17 February 1978—all surviving.*
This case was mentioned in the *Mainichi* newspaper report on the Takeda quads (see below). There were two girls and two boys, and the birth occurred in Osaka. They were said to be 'in good health', but no further details were given.

ANON., *Japan, 16 March 1978—all surviving.*
Another set mentioned in the *Mainichi* newspaper report on the Takeda quads. Born in Yagamuchi, again there were two girls and two boys, all reportedly healthy, but again with no further details.

ANON., *Japan, April 1978—none surviving.*
The third set of Japanese quads mentioned in the *Mainichi* newspaper report on the Takeda quads. The four babies were delivered two months preterm at Kagoshima Municipal Hospital, and all died shortly after birth.

ANON., *South Africa, 29 September 1978—all surviving.*
A 22-year-old Black woman from Durban was referred to hospital at 38 weeks because X-rays had revealed more than one fetal skull. Re-examination of that X-ray showed three heads. Within 12 hours of admission the mother reported the onset of labour and a test provided evidence of fetal lung maturity. Preparations were made for the delivery and a caesarian section was performed. The fourth baby was discovered after the easy birth of the first three. The babies were all girls, with birthweights ranging from 1850 to 1950g. There were four separate placentae with separate amniotic and chorionic sacs. There were some minor problems with the infants but all responded well to treatment. The mother appeared to be relatively undaunted by the sudden increase in her family, apart from understandable concern about the practical problems of coping with so many babies at once. However, publicity in the local paper resulted in the family being rehoused, and a number of gifts were received which helped alleviate some of the initial problems.

Riley, P. (1979) 'Quadruplets delivered by caesarian section.' *South African Medical Journal*, **55**, 3.

TAKEDA, *Japan, 2 October 1978—all surviving.*
This all-girl set is featured in the current *Guinness Book of Records* as the heaviest set ever born, the birthweights being 2350, 2600, 2800 and 2600g respectively, a total of 10,350g (see, however: Norriss, 28 March 1889; Anon., 27 July 1907). The birth took place at the Tsuchihashi Maternity Hospital, Kagoshima, and was reported by the *Mainichi* newspaper (4 October 1978). The translation provided for that article (courtesey Guinness Books) is somewhat enigmatic, stating that 'Dr Tsuchihashi's treatment aimed to hold the delivery until the 10th month to prevent premature birth'; and again, 'Delivery was three weeks earlier than expected, but her pregnancy was already in the 10th month and all four babies are doing well'. Ultrasonography on 17 August had revealed only three fetuses. This was the

31-year-old mother's third pregnancy, and she had not been on fertility drugs. Birth was by vaginal delivery, with only two-minute intervals between each of the babies. To protect them from infection, they were moved to the preterm baby unit at the Kagoshima University Hospital the following day. The first three babies were all of blood group B, Rh+, the last-born being A, Rh+. They were the fourth set of quads born in Japan during 1978.

ANON., *Canada, reported 1979—all surviving.*
This was the 32-year-old mother's second pregnancy, her first child having died from gastroenteritis and septicemia at 3 weeks. When multiple pregnancy was suspected at 16 weeks an ultrasound examination was conducted and the scan confirmed the presence of four fetuses. By 20 weeks the mother's condition had deteriorated considerably and she was admitted to the Women's College Hospital, Toronto. Progress was continuously monitored and in the 31st week it was decided to perform a caesarian section. The infants, all girls, were safely delivered; birthweights were 1390, 1190, 1120 and 1115g. Two required assistance to establish breathing, and later two needed blood transfusions because of interquadruplet transfusion. The blood group of all four was O, Rh+, and the placenta was monochorionic and quadriamniotic, suggesting that the quads constituted an MZ set. Subsequent progress was satisfactory but discharge was delayed until 11 weeks due to the difficulty in finding suitable accommodation for the enlarged family.

Shennan, A.T., Milligan, J.E., Yeung, P.K. (1979) 'Successful management of quadruplet pregnancy in a perinatal unit.' *Canadian Medical Association Journal*, **121**, 741–744.

ROBERSON, *USA, 4 December 1979—all liveborn.*
This birth occurred at the Angelo Community Hospital, San Angelo, TX, and was reported by the *San Angelo Standard Times* (5 December 1979). The 22-year-old mother had been on a course of fertility drugs. Ultrasonography had shown only three fetuses; the fourth infant was only discovered at the birth, which was by caesarian section, two weeks preterm. The babies—four boys—were all of good weight, the lightest being about 2150g.

DALE, *England, 22 January 1980—all surviving at 4 years.*
There was a family history of multiple birth, the mother's father having been one of twins, and her older sister having previously given birth to triplets. The mother had already had one stillborn baby and two miscarriages when these quads were diagnosed by ultrasonographic scan at three months. She was admitted to hospital for the remainder of her pregnancy. No details of the birth were given in the report, published in *You* magazine (15 January 1984), but it was stated that the smallest baby weighed 2 lbs. 4 oz. (about 1020g), and that all the infants 'remained in incubators in the premature-baby ward until their weight climbed above danger level.' There were three girls (Clare, Rachel, Rebecca) and a boy (Andrew). The father worked nights, the mother coping with much help from friends and

neighbours. They live in a three-bedroomed semi-detached house, purchased from the local council.

Despite the overcrowding, her home is as neat as a mail-order catalogue and the quads, now boisterous four-year-olds, are impeccably well-behaved. They have a fierce sense of sibling loyalty, so that if Gail [the mother] chastises one, the other three instantly take the villain's side, cooing words of comfort and understanding, and making Gail 'feel an absolute heel'.

ASIATA, *Western Samoa (birth in New Zealand), 1 July 1980—all surviving.*
Details of this birth were provided by Professor D.G. Bonham of the National Women's Hospital, Auckland *(personal communication)*. The mother, aged 20 years with one previous pregnancy and a 2-year-old son, lived in a village in Western Samoa. Quadruplets were diagnosed by X-ray at around 20 to 22 weeks gestation and at 33 weeks she was flown to New Zealand for the confinement. The babies (all girls) were delivered by caesarian section four minutes apart. There was a single placenta and extensive blood testing supported the view that they were an MZ set. Despite being born preterm, their condition at birth was good and they were soon 'screaming their heads off'. Birthweights ranged from 1810 to 2020g, with a total weight of 7350g. Apparently the mother breast-fed them all. They were discharged from the hospital at 8 weeks.

The family stayed on in New Zealand after the birth. A report in the *New Zealand Herald* (28 June 1983) stated that the quads were returning to Western Samoa for their third birthday.

PETER, *Tanzania, 16 December 1980—all surviving at 11 months.*
The mother was 38 years old and had eight children already. She was first seen at the medical missionary clinic in September. On palpation she was thought to have a multiple pregnancy and she was admitted to hospital for bed-rest. X-ray examination indicated the presence of quads. Contractions began at 6am on 16th December. After 13 hours of labour in the first stage and 20 minutes in the second she gave birth to two boys and two girls with birthweights of 2750, 2000, 1880 and 1700g. The first two placentae expelled were separate and the last two were accompanied by a single amniotic sac. Mid-way through the birth the hospital's generator failed and all the lights went out; they proceeded by torch-light until lamps could be lit. The report gives details of nursing care, nutrition and medication given.

The medical staff were anxious to keep the babies in hospital until they were all at least 2500g, but the father continually asked to take them home. This was about 60km away and it was felt that they would be unable to obtain sufficient milk supplies. However, on 5th February both mother and babies went missing. The father had taken them to a nearby house, but as he had no milk to feed them he brought them back again that evening. Soon after this he rented a room for his family near to the hospital so as to have access to food for the babies. At 11 months all the infants were well, crawling and using their first words.

Aherne, H. (1983) 'Multiple birth.' *Nursing Times,* **79** (50), 36–37.

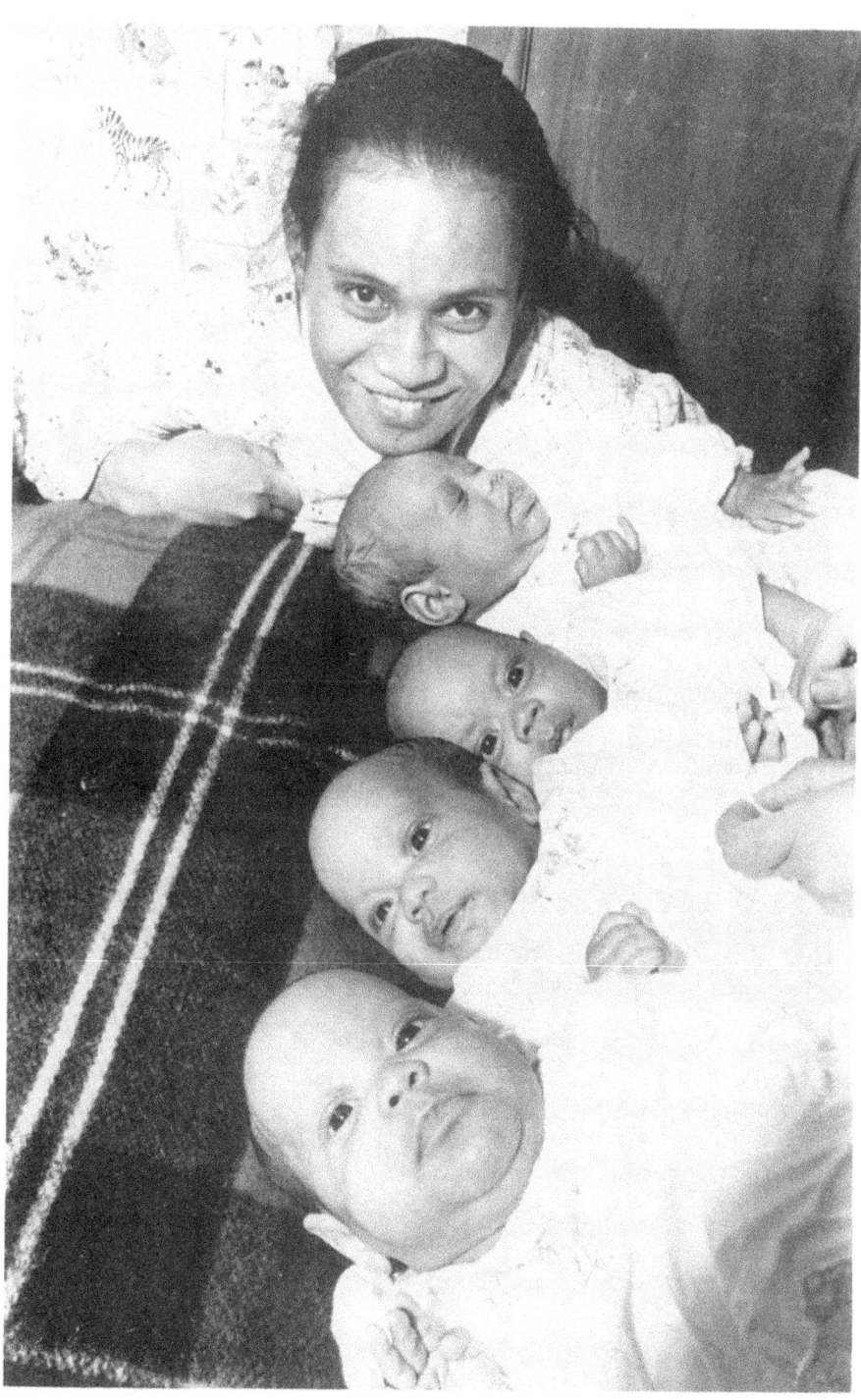

The **Asiata** quads (photo: *New Zealand Herald*)

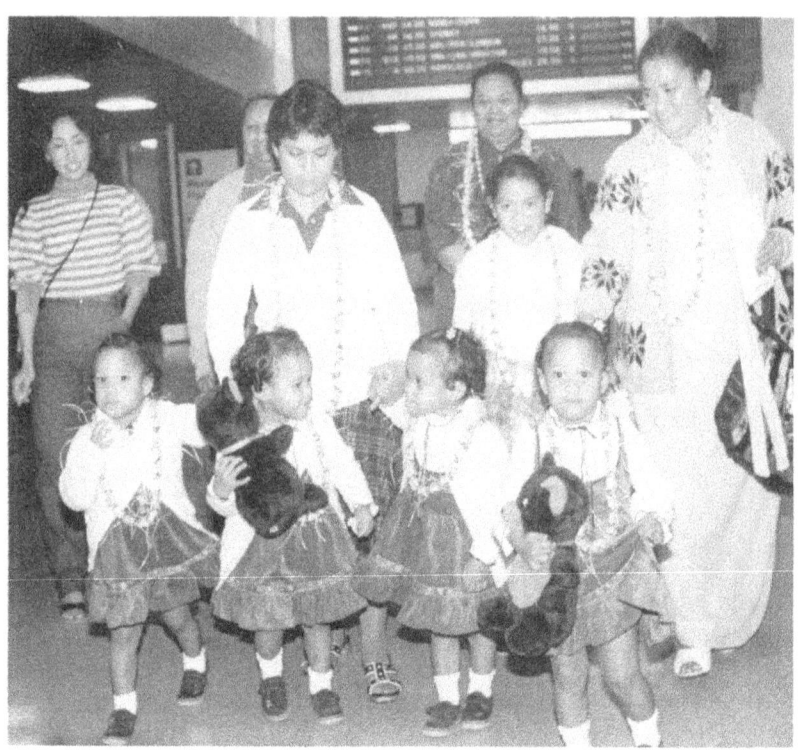

The **Asiata** quads (*l–r*, Pato, Lise, Lakena, Tuaula) with their mother and other relatives at Auckland International Airport, *en route* to Western Samoa to celebrate their third birthday (photo: *New Zealand Herald*)

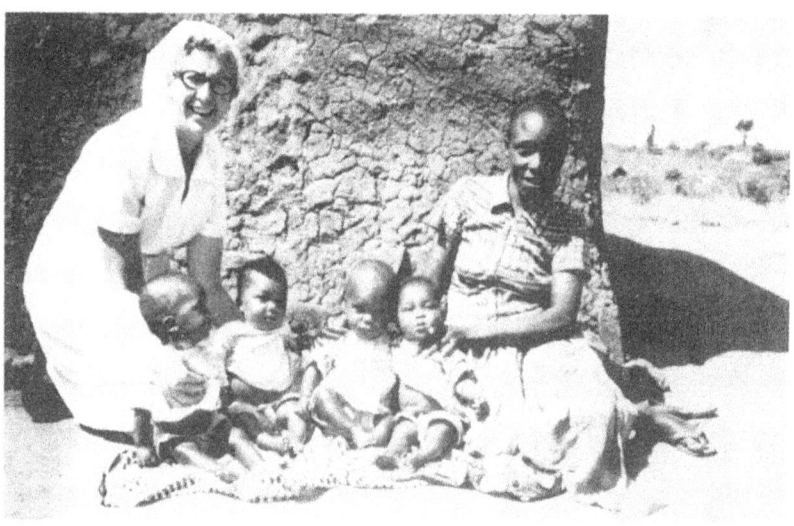

The **Peter** quads with their mother and Sister Helen Aherne, author of the case report (photo reproduced by kind permission of the *Nursing Times*)

ANON., *Reported 1980, no birth details—all surviving at 2 years.*
The first two years of development of quads born after fertility treatment were reported. No details of family or prenatal history were given. The quads, who were delivered at 31 weeks gestational age, were kept in incubators for between 11 and 21 days, and were discharged at 2 to 3 weeks.

Krall, V., Feinstein, S., Kennedy, D. (1980) 'Birth weight and measures of development, object constancy, and attachment in multiple birth infants: a brief report.' *International Journal of Behavioral Development*, **3**, 501–505.

WAGNER, *USA, 6 April 1981—all surviving at 14 months.*
Another of the sets of quads included in the gathering for the *Guinness Book of World Records* on 5 June 1982 (see Struve, 12 June 1974). An all-male set (Chad, Ben, Kyle and Brett).

CLAY, *England, 10 May 1981—all surviving at 5 years.*
A set comprising three boys (Philip, Benjamin, Timothy) and one girl (Victoria). They were born by caesarian section at the University College Hospital, London, the delivery taking only two minutes (information courtesy Guinness Books). The *Cambridge Evening News* (9 April 1986) reported their first day at school.

MEDINA, *USA, 20 September 1981—all surviving at 8 months.*
The youngest of the four sets of quads who took part in the record-breaking assembly of triplets and quads arranged by the *Guinness Book of World Records* on 5 June 1982 (see Struve, 12 June 1974). On the record sheet detailing the participants, their names are given as Kelly, Ragina, Mitchel and Shain, but as the first of those names is used as both a boy's and a girl's name, the sex of this child is unclear.

ANON., *USA, 17 December 1981—all surviving.*
The mother, a 26-year-old Caucasian living in Ohio with one daughter, was receiving ovulation induction therapy. At six to eight weeks gestation ultrasonography revealed a quadruplet pregnancy. She was hospitalized at 27 weeks. A caesarian section was performed and four boys were delivered within two minutes without complications. The mother was discharged on the fifth day. All the babies had mild respiratory distress but all had responded well to treatment by the end of the fourth day. Discharge of the babies from hospital was staggered to allow the family to adapt gradually.

Wu, I.H., Kenneweg, W., Langer, A. (1983) 'Successful management of a quadruplet pregnancy.' *Journal of Reproductive Medicine*, **28**, 163–166.

WARNE, *England, 18 January 1982—all surviving at 2 years.*
A report on this set—four girls named Isabel, Olivia, Rebecca and Sarah—was published in *You* magazine (15 January 1984). No birth details were given. The

mother already had a son of 3 years. When she recognized signs of sibling jealousy developing in him, the article reported that 'she took him and a young friend on an exclusive camping holiday to Devon to reinforce motherly solidarity', leaving the quads with their nanny.

CRAWLEY, *England, 20 January 1982—all alive at 7 years.*
The mother had been on a course of fertility treatment due to ovulatory failure. In an interview published in *Mother* magazine, she said that she had been warned of the possibility of a multiple pregnancy, but to expect twins 'at worst'. Her 'delight' at becoming pregnant turned to 'dismay' when she was informed she was carrying triplets, and when this diagnosis was revised to quadruplets she 'went into a state of shock . . . but I didn't have time to digest the news because they were born, by Caesarian, the next morning.' The problem of the uncertainty associated with fertility drugs was highlighted in her comment that 'I love my children dearly [but] if anybody had told us that there was a good chance that we'd wind up with four babies in one go, I'd never have agreed to the treatment.' The infants—two girls (Hazel, Rebecca) and two boys (Craig, Karl)—weighed between 900 and 1250g, and were kept in the special care unit of the hospital for between six and 10 weeks before being allowed home. The mother was also 'horrified by the lack of information available', saying that 'I've yet to find a book that's relevant to our situation.' As publicity officer for her local branch of the Twins and Multiple Births Association (see Appendix 2, p. 172), the article added, she has since written several advice leaflets for parents with quads. In a recent letter to the present writer (PC, *personal communication*) she confirmed that her four children were all thriving, and at 7½ years 'are totally different in looks and temperament'.

IRWIN, *Australia, February 1982—all surviving.*
This birth was reported in the *Australian Women's Weekly* (17 March 1982). The mother already had two teenaged children and following miscarriage was advised to have a course of ovulation stimulant. She began her labour at home in the morning and she was admitted to the Royal Women's Hospital in Brisbane. The babies were born two hours later by caesarian section and in quick succession. There were two boys and two girls with birthweights from 1410 to 1910g. The delivery team were especially well-prepared as they knew that the parents' religious beliefs would not allow blood transfusions to be given. Within hours the babies were off oxygen, out of danger and in a preterm baby ward.

ANON., *England, May 1982—all surviving.*
A set comprising three girls and a boy. A report in the *Sunday People* newspaper (20 April 1986), concerning the parents of these quads, stated that the quads 'weighed only 2 lb 8 oz [approx. 1135g] when they were born after [their mother] took fertility drugs. But they were all bright and healthy when they were sent home from Portsmouth's St Mary's Hospital . . . The quads will be four next month.'

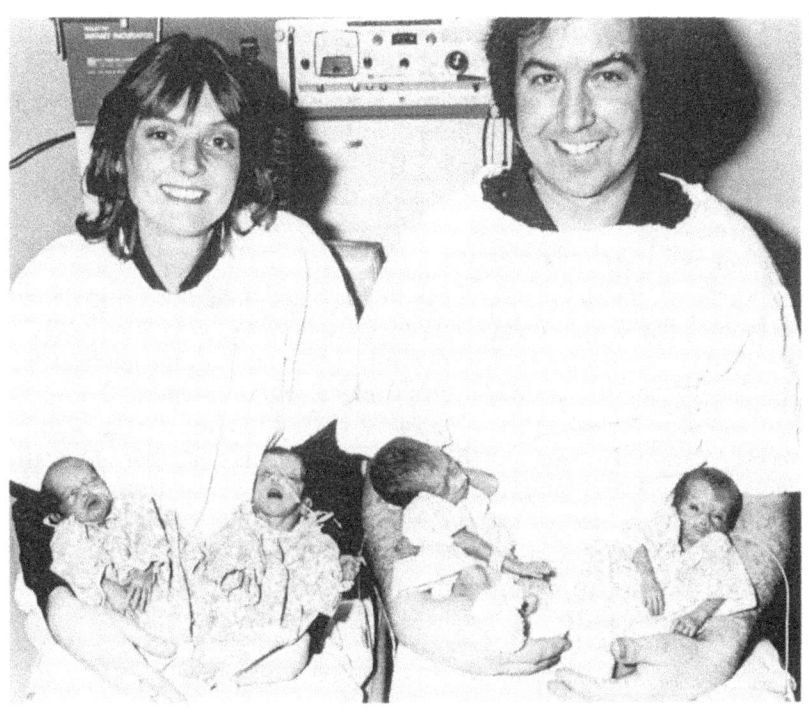

The **Crawley** quads: *above*, four tiny babies provide an 'instant family' for parents Rosemary and Roy Crawley (photo courtesy *The Bucks Herald*); and *below*, aged 3 years (photo reproduced from *Mother* magazine)

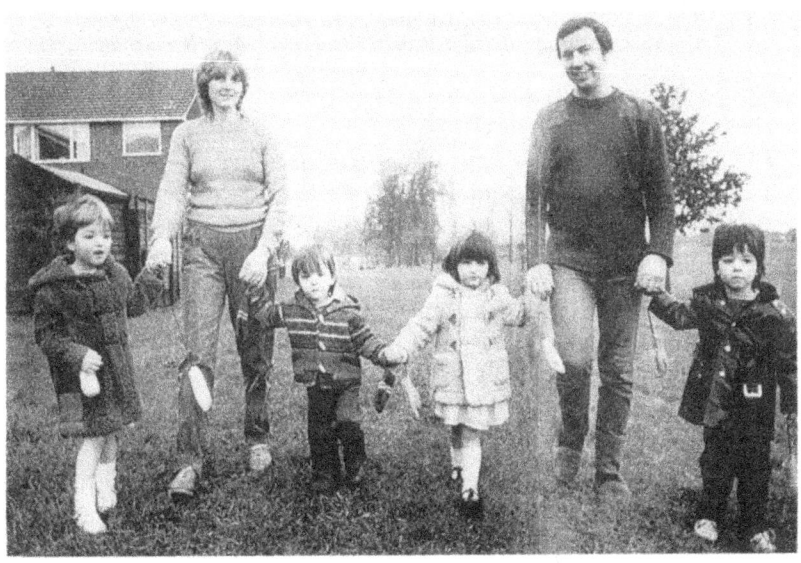

POOLEY, *England, July 1982—all surviving.*
These quads were born at the Rochford Hospital, Essex, with a combined birthweight of 7100g. The mother was 28 years old and already had one son. A photo of mother and babies—Michael, Caroline, Sarah and Victoria—was published in the *New Zealand Women's Weekly* (2 August 1982).

HANE, *Japan, 19 April 1983—all surviving.*
The *New Zealand Herald* (21 April 1983) reported that this all-male set were thought to be of DZ origin, comprising two pairs of MZ 'twins'; however, a later report in the US *National Enquirer* (12 July 1983) stated that medical tests had since established 'that they were identical triplets from one egg and a single brother from another.' The birthweights were 2440, 1985, 1560 and 1500g. The mother, who was 32 years old, lived in Iwamizawa, on Japan's northernmost island of Hokkaido. She had two children already and was not on fertility drugs. Her husband, a farmer, 'told me I was a clever and good wife to provide him with so many fine sons'. The parents asked the island's Governor to think of names for the boys: he chose Akira (meaning 'bright'), Tsuyoshi ('strong'), Makoto ('honest') and Takeshi ('healthy').

ANON., *Japan, reported 1983—all surviving.*
A 28-year-old childless woman received HMG–HCG therapy and conceived quads. Management of her pregnancy involved bed-rest, a salt-restricted diet and administration of β_2 stimulants. Onset of labour occurred at 33 weeks and a caesarian section was performed with successful delivery of babies weighing 1760, 1730, 1590 and 1460g. There was no complications and all four were discharged from hospital at 60 days.

Yamawaki, T., Miyamura, Y., Kawai, Y., Nishimura, K., Uematsu, A., Sugiyama, Y. (1983) 'A quadruplet birth after induced ovulation with HMG–HCG.' *Acta Neonatologica Japonica*, **19**, 186–190.

HAZLETT, *New Zealand, 26 August 1983—all surviving at 4 years.*
The birth and early life of these quads was recorded in several articles published in the *Otago Daily Times* (29 August; 1, 10, 17 September; 22 November 1983). The three girls (Katrina, Melissa, Rochelle) and one boy (Derek) were delivered by caesarian section at the Queen Mary Hospital, Dunedin. The lightest weighed 1130g. The mother came from a farming community in Southland, NZ, and already had one daughter aged 6 years.

MUIR, *Australia, 6 January 1984—all surviving.*
The world's first live-born quadruplets conceived through *in vitro* fertilization were delivered six weeks preterm by caesarian section at the Royal Women's Hospital in Melbourne. The birth was reported by the *New Zealand Herald* (7 January 1984).

The mother was 31 years old and up to this point had been childless. She was given hospital bed-rest for some weeks before the birth, and as she grew larger she was moved to a cooler room with a waterbed. Her four babies were boys weighing 2108, 2071, 1816 and 1775g. The senior paediatrician at the hospital, Dr Neil Roy, told a press conference that he was 'delighted with their condition . . . They are very good weights for babies who have reached 34 weeks and did not seem to be held back in any way by being a multiple birth.' Dr Andrew Spiers, the obstetrician who supervised the delivery, described the mother as 'an ideal patient' who 'never complained', while the father was said to be 'away on planet nine'. In this first report the children's names were given—Sam, Ben, Christopher and Brett—and photographs of the four accompanied the story, but it was stated that the parents 'wish to remain anonymous'. However, a second report in the same newspaper (17 January 1984) named the mother as Mrs Helen Muir, adding that she 'was allowed to return home yesterday, 11 days after giving birth. Doctors said the four boys would leave the Royal Women's Hospital . . . in probably four to five weeks.'

APPENDIX 2

MULTIPLE BIRTH ASSOCIATIONS, SUPPORT GROUPS AND STUDY CENTRES

Australia

Australian Multiple Birth Association,
P.O. Box 105,
Coogee,
NSW 2034

Canada

Parents of Multiple Births Association,
P.O. Box 2200,
Lethbridge,
Alberta T1J 4K7

Eire

Fiona de Buitleir,
Irish Twins Club,
56 Willow Park,
Ennis
Co. Clare

Ethiopa

Ethopian Gemini Trust,
P.O. Box 3547,
Addis Ababa

France

Association d'Enpraide des Parents de Naissances Multiples,
8 Place Alfred Sisley,
95430 Auvers sur Oise

Indonesia

Nakula-sadewa Twin Foundation,
Jl. Teuku Cik Ditiro 32,
Jakarta 10310

Italy

International Society for Twin Studies,
Mendel Institute,
Piazza Galeno 5,
Rome

Japan

Mrs Yukiko Amau,
Minami Aoyama 5 521,
Minato ku,
Tokyo

The Netherlands

Nederlanse Vereniging van Tweelingen,
Jhr Dr J. A. van der Does,
Joh. van Oldenbarneveldlaan 56,
2582 NV Den Haag

New Zealand

New Zealand Multiple Birth Association,
P.O. Box 1258,
Wellington

Nigeria

World-wide Twins and Multiple Births Association,
3 Tiamiyu Street,
Off Ayonuga Street,
Fadeyi Ikorodu Road,
Lagos

South Africa

South African Multiple Births Association,
112 4th Avenue,
Fairland 2195
Johannesburg

United Kingdom

Multiple Births Foundation,
Institute of Obstetrics and Gynaecology Trust,
Queen Charlotte's and Chelsea Hospital,
Goldhawk Road,
London W6 0XG

Study of Triplet and Higher Order Births,
c/o Medical Statistics Division,
Office of Population Censuses and Surveys,
St. Catherine's House,
10 Kingsway,
London WC2B 6JP

Twins and Multiple Births Association,
Jenny Smith,
41 Fortuna Way,
Aylesby Park,
Grimsby,
South Humberside DN37 9SJ

USA

The Center for Study of Multiple Birth,
Suite 476,
333 East Superior Street,
Chicago,
IL 60611

Minnesota Center for Twin and Adoption Research,
Psychology Department,
Elliott Hall,
75 East River Road,
University of Minnesota,
Minneapolis,
MN 55455

National Organization of Mothers of Twins Club, Inc.,
12404 Princess Jeanne N.E.,
Albuquerque,
NM 87112-4640

Twinline,
P.O. Box 10066,
Berkeley,
CA 94709

The Twins Foundation,
P.O. Box 9487,
Providence,
RI 02940-9487

World Multiple Organization,
1120 Linden Drive,
Aurora,
IL 60506

West Germany

ABC-Club,
Strohweg 55,
D-6100 Darmstadt

REFERENCES

Aherne, H. (1983) 'Multiple birth.' *Nursing Times*, **79** (50), 36–37.
Aiken, R.A. (1969) 'An account of the Birmingham "sextuplets".' *Journal of Obstetrics and Gynaecology of the British Commonwealth*, **76**, 684–691.
Allen, G. (1960) 'A differential method for estimation of type frequencies in triplets and quadruplets.' *American Journal of Human Genetics*, **12**, 210–224.
—— Firschein, L.I. (1957) 'The mathematical relations among plural births.' *American Journal of Human Genetics*, **9**, 181–190.
Anastasi, A. (1979) *Fields of Applied Psychology, 2nd Edn.* New York: McGraw-Hill.
Baltes, P.B., Reese, H.W., Nesselroade, J.R. (1977) *Life-span Developmental Psychology: Introduction to Research Methods.* Monterey, CA: Brooks/Cole with Wadsworth.
Bayley, N. (1963) 'Intellectual and physical development.' *In:* Rosenthal, D. (Ed.) *The Genain Quadruplets.* New York: Basic Books.
Berton, P. (1977) *The Dionne Years: A Thirties Melodrama.* New York: Norton.
Beruti, J.A. (1944) 'El parto de los quintigéminos argentinos. Una reconstrucción con datos suministrados por los padres y la partera.' *La Semana Médica*, **51**, 689–696.
Bhargava, I., Chakravarty, A., Raja, P.T.K. (1971) 'An anatomical study of the foetal blood vessels on the chorial surface of the human placenta. Part III. Multiple pregnancies.' *Acta Anatomica*, **80**, 465–479.
Blatz, W.E. (1937) 'Abstracts of studies on the development of the Dionne quintuplets.' *Canadian Medical Association Journal*, **37**, 424–433.
—— (1939) *The Five Sisters: A Study of the Dionne Quintuplets.* New York: William Morrow; London: J.M. Dent.
—— Millichamp, D.A. (1937) 'The mental growth of the Dionne quintuplets.' *In:* Blatz, W.E. (and others) *Collected Studies on the Dionne Quintuplets.* Toronto: University of Toronto Press.
—— Chart, N., Charles, M.W., Fletcher, M.I., Ford, N.H.C., Harris, A.L., MacArthur, J.W., Mason, M., Millichamp, D.A. (1937) *Collected Studies on the Dionne Quintuplets.* Toronto: University of Toronto Press.
—— Fletcher, M.I., Mason, M. (1937a) 'Early development in spoken language of the Dionne quintuplets.' *In:* Blatz, W.E. (and others) *Collected Studies on the Dionne Quintuplets. (Idem.)*
—— Millichamp, D.A., Charles, M.W. (1937b) 'The early social development of the Dionne quintuplets.' *In:* Blatz, W.E. (and others) *Collected Studies on the Dionne Quintuplets. (Idem.)*
Bogdanowicz, M. (1974) 'Psychomotor development of the Danzig quintuplets in their first year of life: a psychological evaluation.' *Acta Geneticae Medicae et Gemellologiae*, **22** (Suppl.), 186–188.
Botting, B.J., MacDonald Davies, I., MacFarlane, A.J. (1987) 'Recent trends in the incidence of multiple births and associated mortality.' *Archives of Disease in Childhood*, **62**, 941–950.
Brattström, E. (1914) 'Ein Fall von viereiigen Vierlingen nebst einigen Beobachtungen betreffs der Vierlingsgeburten in allgemeinen.' *Monatsschrift für Geburtshilfe und Gynäkologie*, **40**, 53–69.
Brintle, S.L. (1931) 'Mental and physical measurements of a set of twelve-year-old quadruplets.' *Journal of Genetic Psychology*, **39**, 91–112.
British Medical Journal (1934) 'The quintuplets.' **2**, 562.
Browne, J.C.McC., Dixon, G. (1978) *Browne's Antenatal Care, 11th Edn.* Edinburgh: Churchill Livingstone.
Brough, J., with the Dionnes (1965) *We Were Five.* New York: Simon & Schuster.
Bryan, E.M. (1983) *The Nature and Nurture of Twins.* London: Baillière Tindall.
Buchsbaum, M.S., Mirsky, A.F., DeLisi, L., Morihisa, J., Karson, C.N., Mendelson, W.B., King, A.C., Johnson, J., Kessler, R. (1984) 'The Genain quadruplets: electrophysiological, positron emission, and X-ray tomographic studies.' *Psychiatry Research*, **13**, 95–108.
Bulmer, M.G. (1958) 'The numbers of human multiple births.' *Annals of Human Genetics*, **22**, 158–164.
—— (1970) *The Biology of Twinning in Man.* (1970) Oxford: Clarendon Press.
Burgoine, E., Wing, L. (1983) 'Identical triplets with Asperger's syndrome.' *British Journal of Psychiatry*, **143**, 261–265.
Burnell, G.M. (1974) 'Maternal reaction to the loss of multiple births. A case of septuplets.' *Archives of General Psychiatry*, **30**, 183–184.
Cadden, V. (1962) 'Crisis in the family.' *Reprinted in:* Caplan, G. (1964) *Principles of Preventive Psychiatry.* London: Tavistock. (Appendix B.)

Cameron, A.H., Robson, E.B., Wade-Evans, T., Wingham, J. (1969) 'Septuplet conception: placental and zygosity studies.' *Journal of Obstetrics and Gynaecology of the British Commonwealth*, **76**, 692–698.
Campbell, D.T., Stanley, J.C. (1963) 'Experimental and quasi-experimental designs for research on teaching.' *In:* Gage, N.L. (Ed.) *Handbook of Research on Teaching.* Chicago: Rand–McNally
Caplan, G. (1961) *An Approach to Community Mental Health.* London: Tavistock.
Carey, H.M. (1976) 'Induction of ovulation resulting in nonuplet pregnancy.' *Australia and New Zealand Journal of Obstetrics and Gynaecology*, **16**, 200–202.
Cederlöf, R., Friberg, L., Jonsson, E., Kaij, L. (1961) 'Studies on similarity diagnosis in twins with the aid of mailed questionnaires.' *Acta Geneticae Medicae et Gemellologiae*, **11**, 338–362.
Clarke, A.E. (1932) 'Identical quadruplets.' *Journal of Heredity*, **23**, 257–259.
Clay, M.M. (1979) *Reading: the Patterning of Complex Behaviour, 2nd Edn.* Auckland: Heinemann.
—— (1982) *Observing Young Readers.* Exeter, NH: Heinemann Educational.
—— (1985) *The Early Detection of Reading Difficulties.* Auckland: Heinemann.
—— Oates, R. (1984) *Round-about Twelve.* University of Auckland Department of Education. (Research report.)
—— Gill, M., Glynn, E., McNaughton, A.H., Salmon, K. (1983) *Record of Oral Language* and *Biks and Gutches.* Auckland: Heinemann.
Cohen, D.J. Dibble, E., Grawe, J.M., Pollin, W. (1973) 'Separating identical from fraternal twins.' *Archives of General Psychiatry*, **29**, 465–469.
—— —— —— —— (1975) 'Reliably separating identical from fraternal twins.' *Archives of General Psychiatry*, **32**, 1371–1375.
Corner, B.D. (1974) 'The Bristol quadruplets: twenty-four year history.' *Acta Geneticae Medicae et Gemellologiae*, **22** (Suppl.), 149–153.
Corney, G., Robson, E.B. (1975) 'Types of twinning and determination of zygosity.' *In:* MacGillivray, I., Nylander, P.P.S., Corney, G. (Eds.) *Human Multiple Reproduction.* Philadelphia: W.B. Saunders.
—— —— Strong, S.J. (1972) 'The effect of zygosity on the birth weight of twins.' *Annals of Human Genetics*, **36**, 45–59.
Cunningham, C.E., Barkley, R.A. (1978) 'The effects of methylphenidate on the mother–child interactions of hyperactive identical twins.' *Developmental Medicine and Child Neurology*, **20**, 634–642.
Dafoe, A.R. (1934) 'The Dionne quintuplets.' *Journal of the American Medical Association*, **103**, 673–677.
—— (1936) 'Further history of the care and feeding of the Dionne quintuplets.' *Canadian Medical Association Journal*, **34**, 26–32.
—— (1940) 'Survival of the Dionne quintuplets.' *American Journal of Obstetrics and Gynecology*, **39**, 159–164.
—— Dafoe, W.A. (1937) 'The physical welfare of the Dionne quintuplets.' *Canadian Medical Association Journal*, **37**, 415–423.
Dahlberg, G. (1926) *Twin Births and Twins from a Hereditary Point of View.* Stockholm: Tidens Tryckeri.
da Silva, B.T., Borges Osorio, M.R.L., Salzano, F.M. (1975) 'School achievement, intelligence and personality in twins.' *Acta Geneticae Medicae et Gemellologiae*, **24**, 213–219.
Day, E.J. (1932) 'The development of language in twins: a comparison of twins and single children.' *Child Development*, **3**, 179–199.
DeFries, J.C., Vandenberg, J.G., McClearn, G.F. (1976) 'Genetics of specific cognitive abilities.' *Annual Review of Genetics*, **10**, 179–207.
DeLisi, L.E., Mirsky, A.F., Buchsbaum, M.S., van Kammen, D.P., Berman, K.F., Caton, C., Kafka, M.S., Ninan, P.T., Phelps, B.H., Karoum, F., Ko, G.N., Korpi, E.R., Linnoila, M., Sheinan, M., Wyatt, R.J. (1984) 'The Genain quadruplets 25 years later: a diagnostic and biochemical followup.' *Psychiatry Research*, **13**, 59–76.
Derom, C., Bakker, E., Vlietinck, R., Derom, R., Van den Berghe, H., Thiery, M., Pearson, P. (1985) 'Zygosity determination in newborn twins using DNA variants.' *Journal of Medical Genetics*, **22**, 279–282.
Dibble, E., Cohen, D.J., Grawe, J.M. (1978) 'Methodological issues in twin research: the assumption of environmental equivalence.' *In:* Nance, W.E., and others (Eds.) *Twin Research: Part A. Psychology and Methodology.* New York: Alan R. Liss.
Drillen, C.M. (1964) *The Growth and Development of the Prematurely-born Infant.* Edinburgh: E. & S. Livingstone.

Duchatel, F., Mennesson, B. (1985) '"Diapolyembryonie" sur septuplés—réduction du nombre d'embryons en début de grossesse.' *Gynécologie*, **36**, 135–140.
Dunkley, P.A. (1967) 'Premature and plural—be prepared.' *New Zealand Nursing Journal* (August), 8–12.
Dziedziuszko, A., Krywko, A. (1974) 'The Danzig quintuplets: perinatal complications and first days of life.' *Acta Geneticae Medicae et Gemellologiae*, **22** (Suppl.), 170–174.
Eaves, L.J. (1972) 'Computer simulation of sample size and experimental design in human psychogenetics.' *Psychological Bulletin*, **77**, 144–152.
—— Eysenck, H. (1975) 'The nature of extraversion: a genetical analysis.' *Journal of Personality and Social Psychology*, **32**, 102–112.
—— —— (1976) 'Genetic and environmental components of inconsistency and unrepeatability in twins' responses to a neuroticism questionnaire.' *Behavior Genetics*, **6**, 145–160.
Edwards, J.H. (1968) 'The value of twins in genetic studies.' *Proceedings of the Royal Society of Medicine*, **61**, 227–229.
Ellis, J.P., Williamson, J.C. (1975) 'Factors influencing the pregnancy and complication rates with human menopausal gonadotropin therapy.' *British Journal of Obstetrics and Gynaecology*, **82**, 52–57.
Elsässer, K. (1906) 'Zur Entstehung von Brady- und Dolichocephalie durch willkürliche Beeinflussung des kindlichen Schädels.' *Zentralblatt für Gynäkologie*, **30**, 422–424.
Eriksson, A.W., Eskola, M.R., Fellman, J.O. (1976) 'Respective studies on the twinning rate in Scandinavia.' *Acta Geneticae Medicae et Gemellologiae*, **25**, 29–35.
Erlenmeyer-Kimling, L. (1975) 'A prospective study of children at risk for schizophrenia.' In: Wirt, R.D., Winokur, G., Roff, M. (Eds.) *Life History Research in Psychopathology*. Minneapolis: University of Minnesota Press.
Fischbein, S. (1977) 'Onset of puberty in MZ and DZ twins.' *Acta Geneticae Medicae et Gemellologiae*, **26**, 151–158.
Foch, T.T., Plomin, R. (1980) 'Specific cognitive abilities in 5- to 12-year-old twins.' *Behavior Genetics*, **10**, 507–520.
Ford, N., Mason, A.D. (1941) 'Taste reactions of the Dionne quintuplets.' *Journal of Heredity*, **32**, 365–368.
—— —— (1943) 'Heredity as an aetiological factor in malocclusion, as shown by a study of the Dionne quintuplets.' *Journal of Heredity*, **34**, 57–64.
Fowler, W. (1965) 'A study of process and method in three-year-old twins and triplets learning to read.' *Genetic Psychology Monographs*, **72**, 3–89.
Fox, H. (1978) *Pathology of the Placenta*. London: W.B. Saunders.
Fullerton, W.T., Hytten, F.E., Klopper, A.I., McKay, E. (1965) 'A case of quadruplet pregnancy.' *Journal of Obstetrics and Gynaecology of the British Commonwealth*, **72**, 791–796.
Galton, F. (1875) 'The history of twins, as a criterion of the relative powers of nature and nurture.' *Journal of the Anthropological Institute of Great Britain and Ireland*, **5**, 391–406.
Gardner, I.C., Newman, H.H. (1940a) 'The alphabetical Perricone quadruplets. A four-egg set, all males.' *Journal of Heredity*, **31**, 307–314.
—— —— (1940b) 'Physical and mental traits of the College Quadruplets.' *Journal of Heredity*, **31**, 418–424.
—— —— (1942) 'Studies of quadruplets. IV. The Badgett quadruplets.' *Journal of Heredity*, **33**, 345–350.
—— —— (1943a) 'Studies of quadruplets. V. The Kaspar quadruplets. *Journal of Heredity*, **34**, 27–32.
—— —— (1943b) 'Studies of quadruplets. V. [sic] The only living one-egg quadruplets.' *Journal of Heredity*, **34**, 258–263.
—— —— (1944) 'Studies of quadruplets. VII. The Schenses, four-egg quadruplets.' *Journal of Heredity*, **35**, 83–88.
Garthshore, M. (1787) 'A remarkable case of numerous births with observations.' *Philosophical Transactions of the Royal Society*, **77**, 344–358.
Gedda, L. (1961) *Twins in History and Science*. Springfield, IL: Charles C. Thomas.
—— (1963) 'On the statistical significance of one pair of monozygotic twins in clinical genetics.' *Acta Geneticae Medicae et Gemellologiae*, **12**, 317–323.
—— (1972) 'Twin studies in genetics.' *Acta Geneticae Medicae et Gemellologiae*, **21**, 265–269.
—— Brenci, G. (1975) 'Twins as a natural test of chronogenetics.' *Acta Geneticae Medicae et Gemellologiae*, **24**, 15–30.
Gemzell, C. (1967) 'The problem of multiple births following treatment with human gonadotropins.' In: Westin, B., Wiqvist, N. (Eds.) *Proceedings of the Fifth World Congress on Fertility and Sterility*. Excerpta Medica International Congress Series No. 133. London: Excerpta Medica Foundation.

Gesell, A., Thompson, H. (1929) 'Learning and growth in identical infant twins.' *Genetic Psychology Monographs*, **6**, 1–124.

—— —— (1941) 'Twins T and C from infancy to adolescence.' *Genetic Psychology Monographs*, **24**, 3–123.

Gillberg, C. (1983) 'Identical triplets with infantile autism and the fragile-X syndrome.' *British Journal of Psychiatry*, **143**, 256–260.

Giovanaucci-Uzielli, M.L., Vecchi, C., Donzelli, G.P., Levi d'Ancona, V., Lapi, E. (1981) 'The history of the Florentine sextuplets: obstetric and genetic considerations.' *In:* Gedda, L., and others (Eds.) *Twin Research 3: Twin Biology and Multiple Pregnancy.* New York: Alan R. Liss.

Glaser (1881) 'Ein Fall von Vierlingsgeburt.' *Correspondenz-Blatz für Schweizer Aerzte*, **11**, 302.

Goshen-Gottstein, E.R. (1976) *Coping Behaviour of Mothers of Multiple Births.* Jerusalem: Centre of Demography, Prime Minister's Office.

—— (1980) 'The mothering of twins, triplets and quadruplets.' *Psychiatry*, **43**, 189–204.

Gottesman, I.I. (1963) 'Genetic aspects of intelligent behavior.' *In:* Ellis, N.R. (Ed.) *Handbook of Mental Deficiency.* New York: McGraw–Hill.

—— (1965) 'Personality and natural selection.' *In:* Vandenberg, S.G. (Ed.) *Methods and Goals in Human Behavior.* New York: Academic Press.

Green, G.H. (1967) 'Multiple pregnancy.' *New Zealand Nursing Journal*, (August), 5–7.

Greulich, W.W. (1930) 'The incidence of human multiple births.' *American Naturalist*, **64**, 142–153.

Gutowitz, H.E., Baillie, P., Harrison, V., Zief, S. (1974) 'Sextuplet gestation: a case report.' *South African Medical Journal*, **48**, 1449–1452.

Guttmacher, A.F. (1953) 'The incidence of multiple births in man and some of the other unipara.' *Obstetrics and Gynecology*, **2**, 22–35.

Hafez, E.S.E. (1974) 'Physiology of multiple pregnancy.' *Journal of Reproductive Medicine*, **12**, 88–96.

Hamilton, W.J., Brown, D., Spiers, B.G. (1959) 'Another case of quadruplets.' *Journal of Obstetrics and Gynaecology of the British Empire*, **66**, 409–412.

Hamlett, G.W.D. (1935) 'Human twinning in the United States: racial frequencies, sex ratios, and geographical variations.' *Genetics*, **20**, 250.

Harrison, E.H. (1935) 'The Eynesbury quadruplets.' *British Medical Journal*, **1**, 1207–1208.

Hathaway, S.R., McKinley, J.C. (1951) *Minnesota Multiphasic Personality Inventory: Manual.* New York: Psychological Corporation.

Hay, D.A., O'Brien, P.J. (1981) 'The interaction of family attitudes and cognitive abilities in the La Trobe twin study of behavioral and biological development.' *In:* Gedda, L., and others (Eds.) *Twin Research 3: Intelligence, Personality and Development.* New York: Alan R. Liss.

—— —— (1984) 'The role of parental attitudes in the development of temperament in twins at home, school, and in test situations.' *Acta Geneticae Medicae et Gemellologiae*, **33**, 191–204.

Hellin, D. (1895) *Die Ursache der Multiparität der Unipaaren Tiere Überhaupt und der Zwillingsschwangerschaft beim Menschen insbesondere.* Munich: Seitz & Schauer.

Henderson, N.D. (1975) 'Gene-environment interaction in human behavioral development.' *In:* Schaie, K.W., Anderson, V.E., McClearn, G.E., Money, J. (Eds.) *Developmental Human Behavior Genetics.* Lexington, MA: D.C. Heath.

Hersen, M., Barlow, D. (1976) *Single Case Experimental Designs: Strategies for Studying Behavior Change.* New York: Pergamon Press.

Hilgard, J.R. (1933) 'The effect of early and delayed practice on memory and motor performances studied by the method of co-twin control.' *Genetic Psychology Monographs*, **14**, 493–667.

Hill, A.V.S., Jeffreys, A.J. (1985) 'Use of minisatellite DNA probes for determination of twin zygosity at birth.' *Lancet*, **2**, 1394–1395.

Husén, T. (1959) *Psychological Twin Research.* Stockholm: Almqvist & Wiksell.

Imaizumi, Y., Inouye, E. (1979) 'Analysis of multiple birth rates in Japan. I: Secular trend, maternal age effect, and geographical variation in twinning rates.' *Acta Geneticae Medicae et Gemellologiae*, **28**, 107–124.

James, W.H. (1972) 'Secular changes in dizygotic twinning rates.' *Journal of Biosocial Science*, **4**, 427–434.

Jarvik, L.F. (1975) 'Commentary II.' (*on:* Harrison, G.A. 'Populations for the study of human behavior traits.') *In:* Schaie, K.W., Anderson, V.E., McClearn, G.E., Money, J. (Eds.) *Developmental Human Behavior Genetics.* Lexington, MA: D.C. Heath.

—— Falek, A. (1961) 'Cancer rates in aging twins.' *American Journal of Human Genetics*, **13**, 413–422.

Jenkins, R.L. (1927) 'Twin and triplet birth ratios.' *Journal of Heredity*, **18**, 387–394.

Jewelewicz, R. (1975) 'Management of infertility resulting from anovulation.' *American Journal of Obstetrics and Gynecology*, **122**, 909–920.

Kaminska, M. (1974) 'Physical development of the Danzig quintuplets in their first year of life.' *Acta Geneticae Medicae et Gemellologiae*, **22** (Suppl.), 178–185.
Kanhai, H.H.H., van Rijssel, E.J.C., Meerman, R.J., Bennebroek Gravenhorst, J. (1986) 'Selective termination in quintuplet pregnancy during first trimester.' *Lancet*, **1**, 1447. *(Letter.)*
Kasriel, J., Eaves, L. (1976) 'The zygosity of twins: further evidence of the agreement between diagnosis by blood groups and written questionnaires.' *Journal of Biosocial Science*, **8**, 263–266.
Keast, A.C., Cooper, G.A. (1967) 'The Tukutese quintuplets.' *South African Journal of Obstetrics and Gynaecology*, **5**, 43–48.
Keettel, W.C. (1941) 'An hitherto unreported case of quintuplet births, Wisconsin, 1875.' *Western Journal of Surgery*, **49**, 636–637.
Kirk, S., McCarthy, J.J., Kirk, W.D. (1968) *The Illinois Test of Psycholinguistic Abilities*. Chicago: University of Illinois Press.
Koch, H.L. (1966) *Twins and Twin Relations*. Chicago: University of Chicago Press.
Krall, V., Feinstein, S., Kennedy, D. (1980) 'Birthweight and measures of development, object constancy and attachment in multiple birth infants: a brief report.' *International Journal of Behavioral Development*, **3**, 501–505.
Kratochwill, T.R. (1978) *Single Subject Research: Strategies for Evaluating Change*. New York: Academic Press.
Lenneberg, E.H. (1966) 'The natural history of language.' *In:* Smith, F., Miller, G. (Eds.) *The Genesis of Language: a Psycholinguistic Approach*. Cambridge, MA: M.I.T. Press.
Levi d'Ancona, V., Coronella, L., Galligani, R., Seravalli, G., Pannuti, P. (1982) 'The Florence sextuplets. Report of a case.' *Acta Europaea Fertilitatis*, **13**, 19–23; 25–34.
Lewontin, R.C. (1975) 'Genetic aspects of intelligence.' *Annual Review of Genetics*, **9**, 387–407.
Ljung, B-O., Fischbein, S., Lindgren, G. (1977) 'A comparison of growth in twins and singleton controls of matched age followed longitudinally from 10 to 18 years.' *Annals of Human Biology*, **4**, 405–415.
Loehlin, J.C. (1975) 'Empirical methods in quantitative human behavior genetics.' *In:* Schaie, K.W., Anderson, V.E., McClearn, G.E., Money, J. (Eds.) *Developmental Human Behavior Genetics*. Lexington, MA: D.C. Heath.
Luria, A.R., Yudovich, F.Ya. (1978) *Speech and the Development of Mental Processes in the Child*, 2nd Edn. Harmondsworth: Penguin.
MacArthur, J.W. (1938) 'Genetics of quintuplets. I. Diagnosis of the Dionne quintuplets as a monozygotic set.' *Journal of Heredity*, **29**, 322–329.
—— Ford, N. (1937) 'A biological study of the Dionne quintuplets—an identical set.' *In:* Blatz, W.E., (and others) *Collected Studies on the Dionne Quintuplets*. Toronto: University of Toronto Press.
—— Dafoe, A.R. (1939) 'Genetics of quintuplets. II. Trends of growth in the Dionne quintuplets.' *Journal of Heredity*, **30**, 359–364.
McDaniel, W.B. (1942) 'An illustrated broadside of 1566 announcing the birth of quintuplets.' *Annals of Medical History*, **4**, 450–452.
McFee, J.G., Lord, E.L., Jeffrey, R.L., O'Meara, O.P., Josepher, H.J., Butterfield, L.J., Thompson, H.E. (1974) 'Multiple gestations of high fetal number.' *Obstetrics and Gynecology*, **44**, 99–106.
McKeown, T., Record, R.G. (1952) 'Observations on foetal growth in multiple pregnancy in man.' *Journal of Endocrinology*, **8**, 386–401.
—— —— (1953) 'The influence of placental size on foetal growth in man, with special reference to multiple pregnancy.' *Journal of Endocrinology*, **9**, 418–426.
Marceil, J.C. (1977) 'Implicit dimensions of idiography and nomothesis: a reformulation.' *American Psychologist*, **32**, 1046–1055.
Martin, N.G., Eaves, L.J. (1977) 'The genetical analysis of covariance structure.' *Heredity*, **38**, 79–95.
Mayer, C.F. (1952a) 'Sextuplets and higher multiparous births. A critical review of history and legend from Aristoteles to the 20th century. Part I. Multiparity and sextuplets.' *Acta Geneticae Medicae et Gemellologiae*, **1**, 118–135.
—— (1952b) 'Sextuplets and higher multiparous births. Part II. Septuplets and higher births.' *Acta Geneticae Medicae et Gemellologiae*, **1**, 242–275.
Metler, S., Rudzinski, J. (1974) 'The Danzig quintuplets: course of gestation.' *Acta Geneticae Medicae et Gemellologiae*, **22** (Suppl.), 161–163.
—— Meyer, J., Rudzinski, L. (1974) 'Morphology of the afterbirth of the Danzig quintuplets.' *Acta Geneticae Medicae et Gemellologiae*, **22** (Suppl.), 164–167.
Metropolitan Life Insurance Co. (1944) *Statistical Bulletin of the Metropolitan Life Insurance Co.*, **25**, 1–2.
Miettinen, M. (1954) 'On triplets and quadruplets in Finland.' *Acta Paediatrica*, **43** (Suppl. 99),

60–61; 76–77.
—— Grönroos, J.A. (1965) 'A follow-up study of Finnish triplets.' *Annales Paediatriae Fenniae*, **11**, 71–83.
Mirenva, A.N. (1935) 'Psychomotor education and the general development of pre-school children.' *Pedagogical Seminary and Journal of Genetic Psychology*, **46**, 433–454.
Mirsky, A.F., DeLisi, L.E., Buchsbaum, M.S., Quinn, O.W., Schwerdt, P., Siever, L.J., Mann, L., Weingartner, H., Zec, R., Sostek, A., Alterman, I., Revere, V., Dawson, S.D., Zahn, T.P. (1984) 'The Genain quadruplets: psychological studies.' *Psychiatry Research*, **13**, 77–93.
Mittler, P. (1969) *Psycholinguistic skills in Four-year-old Twins and Singletons*. Unpublished PhD thesis, University of London.
—— (1971) *The Study of Twins*. Harmondsworth: Penguin.
Mountjoy, P.T. (1957) 'The effects of exposure time and intertrial interval upon rates of decrement in the Müller–Lyer illusion.' *Dissertation Abstracts*, **17**, 2322.
Murphy, M., Botting, B. (1989) 'Twinning rates and social class in Great Britain.' *Archives of Disease in Childhood*, **64**, 272–274.
Myrianthopoulos, N.C. (1975) *Congenital Malformations in Twins: Epidemiologic Survey. Birth Defects Original Articles Series XI: No. 8*. New York: National Foundation March of Dimes.
Newman, H.H. (1940) *Multiple Human Births. Twins, Triplets, Quadruplets and Quintuplets*. New York: Doubleday.
—— (1942) *Twins and Supertwins: A Study of Twins, Triplets, Quadruplets and Quintuplets. Advancement of Science Series No. 1*. London: Hutchinson.
Nichols, J.B. (1950) 'Quintuplets and fecundity.' *Medical Annals of the District of Columbia*, **19**, 601–659.
—— (1952) 'Statistics of births in the United States.' *American Journal of Obstetrics and Gynecology*, **64**, 376–381.
—— (1954) 'Quintuplet and sextuplet births in the U.S.' *Acta Geneticae Medicae et Gemellologiae*, **3**, 143–152.
Nowakowski, T.K. (1974) 'Uniovular quadruplets of Wroclaw.' *Acta Geneticae Medicae et Gemellologiae*, **22** (Suppl.), 154–158.
Nylander, P.P.S. (1969) 'The value of the placenta in the determination of zygosity—a study of 1,052 Nigerian twin maternities.' *Journal of Obstetrics and Gynaecology of the British Commonwealth*, **76**, 699–704.
—— (1971) 'The incidence of triplets and higher multiple births in some rural and urban populations in Western Nigeria.' *Annals of Human Genetics*, **34**, 401–415.
—— (1975) 'The causation of twinning.' *In:* MacGillivray, E., Nylander, P.P.S., Corney, G. (Eds.) *Human Multiple Reproduction*. Philadelphia: W.B. Saunders.
Office of Population Censuses and Surveys (1984) *Multiple Births Series FM1, No. 13*. London: OPCS.
Ounsted, M., Ounsted, C. (1973) *On Fetal Growth Rate. Clinics in Developmental Medicine No. 46*. London: Spastics International Medical Publications with Heinemann Medical.
Overton, W.F. (1973) 'On the assumptive base of the nature–nurture controversy: additive versus interactive conceptions.' *Human Development*, **16**, 74–89.
Pearson, H.A., Grello, F.W., Cone, T.E. (1963) 'Leukemia in identical twins.' *New England Journal of Medicine*, **268**, 1151–1156.
Petri, E. (1935) 'Untersuchungen zur Erbbebingtheit der Menarche.' *Zeitschrift für Morphologie und Anthropologie*, **33**, 43–48.
Pinard, M. (1920) 'Gestation et accouchement quadruples: enfants viables.' *Bulletin de l'Académie de Médecine*, **83**, 169–173.
Placek, P.J., Taffel, S., Moien, M. (1983) 'Cesarian section delivery rates: US, 1981.' *American Journal of Public Health*, **73**, 861–862.
Plomin, R., Willerman, L. (1975) 'A co-twin control study and a twin study of reflection–impulsivity in children.' *Journal of Educational Psychology*, **67**, 537–543.
Potter, A.M., Taitz, L.S. (1972) 'Turner's syndrome in one of MZ twins with mosaicism.' *Acta Paediatrica Scandinavica*, **61**, 473–476.
Potter, E.L. (1963) 'Twin zygosity and placental form in relation to the outcome of pregnancy.' *American Journal of Obstetrics and Gynecology*, **87**, 566–577.
Price, B. (1950) 'Primary biases in twin studies: a review of prenatal and natal difference producing factors in monozygotic pairs.' *American Journal of Human Genetics*, **2**, 293–352.
Price, F.V. (1988) 'Risk of high multiparity with IVF/ET.' *Birth*, **15**, 157–163.
Pryor, J.W. (1936) 'Ossification as additional evidence in differentiating identical and fraternals in multiple births.' *American Journal of Anatomy*, **59**, 409–423.

—— (1939) 'Normal variations in the ossification of bones due to genetic factors.' *Journal of Heredity*, **30**, 248–255.
—— (1948) 'Badgett quadruplets.' *Journal of Heredity*, **39**, 79–84.
Raszeja, S., Krueger, A. (1974) 'Genealogical blood-group analyses of the Danzig quintuplets.' *Acta Geneticae Medicae et Gemellologiae*, **22** (Suppl.), 168–169.
Record, R.G., McKeown, T., Edwards, J.H. (1970) 'An investigation of the differences in measured intelligence between twins and single births.' *Annals of Human Genetics*, **34**, 11–20.
Riekhof, P.L., Horton, W.A., Harris, D.J., Schimke, R.N. (1972) 'Monozygotic twins with the Turner syndrome.' *American Journal of Obstetrics and Gynecology*, **112**, 59–61.
Rife, D.C. (1938) 'Contributions of the 1937 National Twins' Convention to research.' *Journal of Heredity*, **29**, 83–89.
—— Price, B., Snyder, P. (1938) 'Twin light on nature versus nurture. A review of *Twins*.' *Journal of Heredity*, **29**, 21–26.
Robinson, P.W., Foster, D.F. (1979) *Experimental Psychology: A Small-N Approach*. New York: Harper & Rowe.
Rose, J.A. (1961) 'The prevention of mothering breakdown associated with physical abnormalities of the infant.' *In:* Caplan, G. (Ed.) *Prevention of Mental Disorders in Children*. London: Tavistock.
Rosenthal, D. (Ed.) (1963) *The Genain Quadruplets*. New York: Basic Books.
Salisbury, D.M., Jones, R.W.A., Townshend, P., Baum, J.D. 'Paediatric preparation for premature multiple births.' *Early Human Development*, **1**, 39–45.
Scarr-Salapatek, S. (1971) 'Race, social class and I.Q.' *Science*, **174**, 1285–1295.
Schaie, K.W. (1975) 'Research strategy in developmental behavior genetics.' *In:* Schaie, K.W., Anderson, V.E., McClearn, G.E., Money, J. (Eds.) *Developmental Human Behavior Genetics*. Lexington, MA: D.C. Heath.
—— (1977) 'Toward a stage theory of adult cognitive development.' *International Journal of Aging and Human Development*, **8**, 129–138.
Schatz, F. (1882) 'Eine besondere Art von einseitiger Polyhydramnie mit anderseitiger Oligohydramnie bei eineiigen Zwillingen (Makrocardii).' *Archiv für Gynäkologie*, **19**, 329–369.
Scheinfeld, A. (1952) *The New You and Heredity*. London: Chatto & Windus.
—— (1968) *Twins and Supertwins*. London: Chatto & Windus.
—— (1973) *Your Heredity and Environment*. London: Chatto & Windus.
Schenker, J.G., Yarkani, S., Granat, M. (1981) 'Multiple pregnancies following induction of ovulation.' *Fertility and Sterility*, **35**, 105–123.
Schinzel, A.A.G.L., Smith, D.W., Miller, J.R. (1979) 'Monozygotic twinning and structural defects.' *Journal of Pediatrics*, **95**, 921–930.
Schlaginhaufen, O. (1940) 'Die Vierlingsgeschwister Gehri und ihr Verwandtschaftskreis. Eine Familienanthropologische Untersuchung.' *Archiv der Julius Klaus-Stiftung für Vererbungsforschung, Sozialanthropologie und Rassenhygiene*, **15**, 309–398.
Schwesinger, G.C. (1940) 'Five little Dionnes and how they grew.' *Journal of Heredity*, **31**, 145–150.
Scottish Council for Educational Research (1953) *Social Implications of the 1947 Scottish Mental Survey*. London: University of London Press.
Senn, M.J.E. (1975) 'Insights on the child development movement in the United States.' *Monographs of the Society for Research in Child Development*, **40**. (3–4).
Serreyn, R., Thiery, M., Vandekerckhove, D. (1984) 'Outcome of an octuplet pregnancy.' *Archives of Gynecology*, **234**, 283–293.
Shepherd, H.L., Potter, M.F. (1949) 'The quadruplets: 1. Delivery.' *Bristol Medico-Chirurgical Journal*, **66**, 14–16.
Shields, J. (1962) *Monozygotic Twins Brought Up Apart and Brought Up Together*. Oxford: Oxford University Press.
Smith, N.W. (1976) 'Twin studies and heritability.' *Human Development*, **19**, 65–68.
Spier, L. (1928) 'Measurements of quadruplet girls.' *American Journal of Physical Anthropology*, **12**, 269–272.
Spillman, J.R. (1987) 'Emotional aspects of experiencing a multiple birth.' *Midwife, Health Visitor and Community Nurse*, **23**, 54–58.
Stewart, P. (1982) 'Early diagnosis of multiple births.' *Medical Journal of Australia*, **1**, 287. (*Letter*.)
Stocks, P. (1952) 'Recent statistics of multiple births in England and Wales.' *Acta Geneticae Medicae et Gemellologiae*, **1**, 8–13.
Strayer, L.E. (1930) 'Language and growth: the relative efficacy of early and deferred language training studied by the method of co-twin control.' *Genetic Psychology Monographs*, **8**, 209–319.
Strong, S.J., Corney, G. (1967) *The Placenta in Twin Pregnancy*. Oxford: Pergamon Press.

Terman, L.M. (1925) *Genetic Studies of Genius. Vol. 1. Medical and Physical Traits of a Thousand Gifted Children.* Stanford, CA: Stanford University Press.
—— (1954) 'The discovery and encouragement of exceptional talent.' *American Psychologist*, **9**, 221–230.
—— Merrill, M.A. (1937) *Measuring Intelligence: A Guide to the Administration of the Stanford–Binet Tests of Intelligence.* Boston, MA: Houghton Mifflin.
—— —— (1960) *Stanford–Binet Intelligence Scale: Manual for the 3rd Revision, Form L-M.* Boston, MA: Houghton Mifflin.
Thorpe, L.P., Willis, W.C., Tiegs, E.W. (1953) *California Test of Personality: Grades Kindergarten–3.* New York: McGraw-Hill.
Tisserand-Perrier, M. (1953) 'Étude comparative de certains processus de croissance chez les jumeaux.' *Journal de Genetique Humaine*, **2**, 87–102.
Tunnel, G.B. (1977) 'Three dimensions of naturalness: an expanded definition of field research.' *Psychological Bulletin*, **84**, 426–437.
Turksoy, R.N., Toy, B.L., Rogers, J., Papageorge, W. (1967) 'Birth of septuplets following human gonadotropin administration in Chiari–Frommel syndrome.' *Obstetrics and Gynecology*, **30**, 692–698.
United States of America: Bureau of the Census (1942) *Vital Statistics of the United States, Part I.* US Department of Commerce.
VaFai, J., Shapiro, D.L. (1985) 'Perinatal aspects of high multiple gestation.' *New York State Journal of Medicine*, **85**, 560–562.
Vandenberg, S.G. (1968) 'The contribution of twin research to psychology.' *Psychological Bulletin*, **66**, 327–352.
—— Stafford, R.E., Brown, A.M. (1968) 'The Louisville twin study.' In: Vandenberg, S.G. (Ed.) *Progress in Human Behavior Genetics.* Baltimore, MD: Johns Hopkins Press.
Van den Daele, L. (1974) 'Natal influences and twin differences.' *Journal of Genetic Psychology*, **124**, 41–60.
Vaudescal, M.M., Blechmann, G., Levesque, A. (1948) 'Grossesse quadrigemellaire.' *Gynécologie et Obstétrique*, **47**, 883–887.
Vernon, P.E. (1960) *Intelligence and Attainment Tests.* London: University of London Press.
Walcher, G. (1905) 'Über die Entstehung von Brachy- und Dolicocephalie durch willkürliche Beeinflussung des kindlichen Schädels.' *Zentralblatt für Gynäkologie*, **29**, 193–196.
Walker, N.F. (1947) 'A further description of a set of quadriovular quadruplets. (A study of dermal configurations and tooth eruption.)' *American Journal of Obstetrics and Gynecology*, **54**, 266–272.
—— (1950) 'Determination of the zygosity of the Waddington quintuplets born in 1786.' *American Journal of Human Genetics*, **2**, 353–360.
Wechsler, D. (1949) *Wechsler Intelligence Scale for Children: Manual.* New York: Psychological Corporation.
Wilson, J.R., deFries, J.C., McClearn, G.E., Vandenberg, S.G., Johnson, R.C., Rashed, M.M. (1975) 'Cognitive abilities: Use of family data as a control to assess sex and age differences in two ethnic groups.' *International Journal of Aging and Human Development*, **6**, 261–276.
Wilson, P.T. (1934) 'A study of twins with special reference to heredity as a factor determining differences in environment.' *Human Biology*, **6**, 324–354.
Wilson, R.S. (1974) 'Growth standards for twins from birth to four years.' *Annals of Human Biology*, **1**, 175–188.
—— (1977) 'Twins and siblings: concordance for school-age mental development.' *Child Development*, **48**, 211–216.
—— (1979) 'Twin growth: initial deficit, recovery, and trends in concordance from birth to nine years.' *Annals of Human Biology*, **6**, 205–220.
—— Harping, E.B. (1972) 'Mental and motor development in infant twins.' *Developmental Psychology*, **7**, 277–287.
Wyshak, G. (1978) 'Statistical findings on the effects of fertility drugs on plural births.' In: Nance, W.R., and others (Eds.) *Twin Research: Biology and Epidemiology.* New York: Alan R. Liss.
Yoakum, C.S., Yerkes, R.M. (1920) *Army Mental Tests.* New York: Holt.
Young, D. (1973) *Oral Verbal Intelligence Test.* London: Hodder & Stoughton Educational.
Zazzo, R. (1960) *Les Jumeaux: Le Couple et la Personne.* Paris: Presse Universitaire de France.
Zilberman, Y., Robinson, M., Weinstein, D. (1980) 'Clefts in quintuplets: a case report.' *Cleft Palate Journal*, **17**, 58–61.
—— Brin, I., Mahler, D. (1985) 'Quintuplets with clefts: follow-up at 5 years.' *Cleft Palate Journal*, **22**, 205–211.

INDEX

A
abortion
  previous, 35
  selective, 21, 30
  subsequent, 39
abnormality, 27, 31, 89, 98, 104, 109, 115, 141
  concerns about, 36
abuse, as public reaction, 5
adult life, 44–45
advertizing contracts, 38
advice, 10 (plate), 166
  see also information for parents; support groups
Alexander quads, 45, 148–150, 149–150 (photos)
amnion
  definition of, 33 (footnote)
  structure, 33 (fig.), 115
anonymity, 95, 169
attachment links, parent–child, 74–75
'Auckland quads', 42–43, 46
  development
    intelligence, 57, 59 (table), 60 (table)
    language, 57, 65–66, 67 (table)
    reading, 62 (fig.), 63, 68–71, 69–71 (tables)
    visual perception, 57, 59 (figs.)
  digit recall tests, 63
  family relationships, 42–43, 68
  handedness, 55
  personality differences, 73, 74, 74 (fig.)
  school progress, 68–71, 71 (table)
auditory memory, 63
autism, infantile, 75

B
Badgett quads, 4, 39–40, 129 (photo)
  physical characteristics, 50 (table)
behavioural genetics, 88, 91–92
Believe It Or Not (radio series), 19
Bene–Anthony Family Relations Test, 42–43
birth
  caesarian, *see* caesarian section
  Lamaze method, 153
  filming of, 128
  management of, 31
  monitored by closed-circuit TV, 154
  of Dionne quins, 28 (plate)
  order, 91
  preparations for, 31, 158
  preterm, 17, 19, 20, 30, 31
    effect on mental health of mother, 35
  problems, 31–32
  records, importance of keeping, 87
  see also caesarian section
birthweight, 19, 20, 30, 46
  correlation with height, 47 (table)
  correlation with intelligence, 56
  influence of sex and zygosity on, 47
  mean, 46
  metrification, *xii*
  of twins, triplets, quads, 46
  total, 13, 20, 46
    extreme, 13, 104, 108, 152, 155, 160
Blatz, W.E., 1, 25–26
blood
  circulation, mutual, 87, 89
    see also fetofetal transfusion
  cord, samples, 87
  typing, 34, 52, 87, 116, 139, 145
bone ossification, 51–52, 122
Bradlee octuplets, hoax, 17, 18 (plate)
breast-feeding, 40
'Bristol quads', *see* Good quads
Bushnell sextuplets, 19

C
caesarian section, 32
Canada, quadruplet births in, 13
care, 7
cell division, timing, 33 (fig.), 55
child development movement, 23, 24
child rearing, 7, 8
  effect on development, 7
chorion
  definition of, 33 (footnote)
  structure, 33 (fig.), 115
chromosomal anomaly, 32
chronogenetics, 92
circulation, *see* blood
cleft palate
  in quadruplets, 141
  in quintuplets, 75
Coleman sextuplets, 20, 21 (photo)
'College Quadruplets', *see* Keys quads
communication problems, 10
competition between members of set, 42
confidentiality, *xii*, 95
co-twin studies, *see* twin studies
Crawley quads, 36, 166, 167 (photos)
crisis of multiple birth, 35–37

D
Dafoe, Allan Roy, 3, 6 (plate), 28 (plate)
'Danzig quins', 23, 53
  physical development, 54 (fig.)
  psychomotor development, 53–55, 54 (table)
dentition, 52
dermatoglyphics, 32, 128
development
  bone ossification, 51–52
  language, *see* language development
  outcomes, 45
  personal/social, 44

physical, *see* physical development
prenatal, 89
psychological, 25–26
reports, 1, 46–75
diagnosis, 30
differences between MZ sibs, 72, 76, 89–90, 93–94
digit recall, 63, 66
Diligenti quins, 23, 25, 37
Dionne quins, 1, 4, 5 (photo), 5–7, 6 (plate), 8, 21 (footnote), 23, 24, 25–26, 27 (photo), 29 (photos), 37, 46
  birth, 28 (plate)
  development
    cognitive, 91
    language, 64–65 (figs.)
    mental, 57, 58 (figs.)
    physical, 51, 90–91
    psychological, 25–26
  outcomes, 7, 45
  personality differences, 72–73
  publicity, 3, 5–7, 27, 38
  separation from siblings, 42
  television documentary on, 45
  zygosity, 23, 25, 28 (plate)
The Dionne Years: a Thirties Melodrama, 7, 27, 45
DNA probe, 34, 87

E
education, 66–71
  see also school
efficient cause, 88 (footnote)
England and Wales, multiple births in, 13, 15, 16 (table), 138 (table)
environmental factors
  and MZ dissimilarities, 89–90, 94
  and MZ similarities, 89
  controlled, 7, 9, 76, 78, 93–94
  effects of, 1, 56, 72, 76, 82
  pre- and perinatal, 87–88, 89
  similarity, measure of, 77
  vs. heredity, *see* heredity
  see also genetic–environmental interaction
ethics, 41–42, 87

F
family, 35–45
  effect on, 30
  influences, 91
  relationships, 41–44
  rights, 4, 41–42, 87
  support, 4, 37–40
    commercial, 38, 150
fears, maternal, 36
female quads, preponderance of, 2, 16–17
fertility drugs, *see* infertility treatments
fetal growth, 87
  see also twinning mechanism
fetofetal transfusion, 34, 161
  see also blood circulation, mutual

fetus papyraceus, 19, 87, 116, 118
financial hardship, 37–40
financial support, *see* family support
The Five Sisters (Blatz), 1
frequency, 11
  see also Hellin's approximation; incidence

G
Galton, F., 24, 76
gamete intra-fallopian transfer, *see* GIFT
Gardner and Newman, reports, 4, 49, 89
  Badgett quads, 4, 39–40, 50 (table), 129
  Kaspar quads, 38, 127–128
  Keys quads, 4, 113
  Morlok quads, 25, 37, 42, 43, 44, 50 (table), 72, 119–121
  Perricone quads, 118–119
  Schense quads, 37, 39, 50 (table), 59 (table), 122
Gedda, Luigi, 26, 78, 134
Gehri quads, 2, 13, 14 (photo), 27, 45, 99–102, 100–101 (photos)
Genain quads, 45, 46, 146–147
  intelligence, 56–57, 59 (fig.)
  schizophrenia, 75, 146–147
genetic control, 76, 90–92
  over age of menarche, 92
  over intelligence, 56, 66, 90–91
  over motor development, 52
  over personality formation, 72
  over physical development, 47, 51, 90, 91
    in puberty, 92
  over psychological variables, 92
  over school achievement, 66–67
  over spatial ability, 61
  over visual perception, 57
genetic counselling, 10
genetic–environmental interaction, 8, 25, 91, 92, 93
genetic factors
  control over, 79
  overstressed, 89
  see also heredity
genetic manipulation, 10
genetics, study of, 23, 25, 93
  and intelligence, 56
genetic timing mechanisms, 92
Gesell, Arnold, 24, 42, 67, 72, 73, 79, 80
  see also twins, studies of
gestation, length of, 30, 47
GIFT (gamete intra-fallopian transfer), 13
gifts, *see* family support
Good quads, 27, 38, 43–44, 46, 52, 135–136, 136 (photo)
  developmental outcomes, 45
  physical development, 49, 51 (table)
  school progress, 67
Goshen-Gottstein, E.R., 40–41
group characteristics, 44
'group-of-four' behaviour, 42, 43
growth, physical, *see* physical development

Guinness Book of Records (UK), 20, 95, 155, 160
Guinness Book of World Records (USA), 155, 156 (photo), 159, 165

H
haemorrhage, 31
handedness, 55–56
  in twins, 55 (table)
handwriting, 53, 55
health histories, 52
Hellin's approximation, 11, 12, 15
heredity, 24, 78
  identical, 1, 57
  vs. environment, 7, 25, 76, 88, 90, 91, 92
  see also genetic control; genetic–environmental interaction; genetic factors
hoaxes, 7, 17, 18 (plate)
hormone treatments, *see* infertility treatments
hospital procedures, 158

I
'identical' sibs, not necessarily identical, 72, 76, 89–90, 93–94
incidence
  changes over time, 12–13
  historical, 12
  racial variations, 11–12
  sex ratio, 15–17
  studies, 8, 11–17
infant mortality, *see* mortality, infant
infertility treatments, *xi*, 2, 5, 8, 11, 13, 15, 19, 30, 148–168 *passim*
  see also GIFT; *in vitro* fertilization
information for parents
  paucity of, 36, 166
  see also support groups
insurance
  cover, 40, 147
  company statistics, 15, 40
intelligence, 56–57, 66, 77, 91
  pre- and perinatal factors affecting, 87–88
in vitro fertilization (IVF), 2, 13, 30
  first quads, *xii*, 2, 8, 95, 168–169
  first quins, 2

J
Japan, quadruplet births in, 13
Johnson quads, 27, 45, 124 (photo), 124–125

K
Kaspar quads, 38, 127 (photo), 127–128
Keys quads, 4, 13, 24, 25, 27, 44, 46, 52, 111, 113 (photo), 114 (photo)
  intelligence, 56
  personality trait ratings, 73–74, 73 (table)
  physical development, 47–49, 48 (table)
  school progress, 67 (table)

L
labour, early onset, 46

language development, 63–66, 64–65 (figs.), 67 (table)
lateral inversions, 55, 87, 89
Lawson quins, 43

M
male/female ratio, 15–17
male quads
  monozygotic, 45, 141–142
  rarity of, 2, 16
malformations, *see* abnormality
maternal and infant welfare movement, 23, 24
maternal fears, 36
media attention, *xii*, 2–6
  effect on family, 4
  see also press reports; publicity
menarche, timing of, 92, 136
mental illness, 45, 75, 146–147
methodological advice, 14–15
milk banks, 24, 154
Morlok quads, 24, 25, 37, 42, 43, 44, 119–121, 120 (photos)
  bone ossification, 52
  personality differences, 72
  physical characteristics, 50 (table)
mortality, infant, 13, 15, 17, 24, 30, 105
  leaving smaller multiple group, 21, 39
mothering behaviours, 41, 93
motor development, 52–55
Müller–Lyer task (linear illusion problem), 94
multiparity
  family history of, 102, 110, 125, 161
  maternal history of, 19 (footnote), 39, 107, 123, 147
  see also Vassilyev, Feodor
multiple birth associations, 170–172

N
naming quads, ideas used in, 118, 119, 168
'nature *vs.* nurture', *see* heredity *vs.* environment
neonatal care, *xi*, 158
newspaper reports, *see* press reports
New York Times Index (NYTI), 2, 17, 86
New Zealand, quadruplet births in, 13
nontuplets, 17
normality, 10

O
octuplets, 17
Office of Population Censuses and Surveys (OPCS), 40
  birth data, 15, 16 (table)
ossification of bones, *see* bone ossification
overcrowding *in utero*, 31
ovulation treatments, *see* infertility treatments

P
pairings within sets, 43
Perricone quads, 118–119, 118 (photo)
  bone ossification, 51

personality, 72–74
physical features, similarity, 34, 52
physical development, 46–52, 77, 90–91
　genetic control over, 47, 51
　in puberty, 92
placental analysis, 28, 31, 32, 33
　recommendations for, 87
placentation
　monochorionic, 89
　possibilities in MZ twins, 33 (fig.)
　zygosity determination by, 33, 87
pregnancy
　as crisis, 35
　diagnosis, 30
　environmental factors during, 87, 89
　management, 30, 31
　prenatal risk factors, 30–31
press reports, *xi*, 1, 2, 4, 17, 19, 20 (photo), 21 (photo), 43, 86, 95
　see also hoaxes; media attention; publicity
preterm birth, *see* birth, preterm
probability of multiple conception, 12, 32
psychiatric intervention, 36–37
psychology, 76–94
　interest in multiple births, historical, 23–27
psychosocial support, 37
public interest, *xii*, 2–7, 39, 86
publicity, 2, 4, 36, 40, 113, 129, 150, 160
　reaction to, 7, 27, 95
　see also media attention

Q

quadruplet types, 2, 3 (fig.)
　by sex, among cases in Catalogue, 17 (table)
　female, 2, 16–17
　male, 2, 16
　monochorial/monoamniotic, 31
　see also sex ratio; zygosity
quintuplets, 11–12, 21–23, 22 (fig.), 30, 56
　England and Wales, incidence in, 16 (table)
　see also Danzig quins; Diligenti quins; Dionne quins; Lawson quins; Waddington quins

R

racial variations, 11–12
reading
　behaviour, spatial aspects of, 61–63, 62 (figs.), 81
　progress of Auckland quads, 69–71 (tables), 81
　studies of, 81–82
research
　approaches to, 8–9, 75, 77 (table)
　design issues and interpretation of findings, 88–92
　locating subjects, 86–87
　methods, 76–86
　　individual case studies, 77
　　single-subject designs, 83–84
　　time series designs, 26, 66, 80, 83, 84–85
　　twin studies, 78–82
　　within-subject designs, 83–85

planning, 87
recommendations, 93–94
rights, *see* family rights
risk factors, prenatal, 30–31

S

Schense quads, 37, 39, 121 (photos), 121–122
　bone ossification, 51–52
　intelligence, 57, 59 (fig.)
　personality differences, 72
　physical characteristics, 50 (table)
schizophrenia, 75, 146–147
school
　first day, 2, 20 (photo), 165
　progress, 66–71
　　cumulative, 67–68, 68 (table)
　separation at, 43
　　of Auckland quads, 70–71, 71 (table), 93
　　of Walton sextuplets, 20 (photo)
septuplets, 7, 17, 19
　and higher multiples, historical accounts, 17
　England and Wales, incidence in, 16 (table)
　loss of, maternal reaction to, 19, 36–37
services for family, 37–40
sex ratio among multiple births, 15–17
sex role learning, 44
sextuplets, 8, 12, 19–21
　Bushnell, 19
　Coleman, 20, 21 (photo)
　England and Wales
　　incidence in, 16 (table)
　　surviving, 20, 20–21 (photos)
　historical accounts, 17
　Walton, 20 (photo)
sibling jealousy, 166
sibling loyalty, 162
somatic mutation, 31
spatial ability, 61–63
　sex and age differences, 61 (fig.)
spatial aspects of texts, 61–63, 62 (figs.)
stress, maternal, 36, 41
Studio dei Gemelli (Gedda), 134, 135, 137, 140
study centres, 170–172
Study of Triplet and Higher Order Births, *xi*, 16, 40, 171
superfetation, 19, 158–159
superovulation, as a complication of fertility drugs, 13
superstition, 6, 17, 145
support
　financial, 37–40
　psychosocial, 37
support groups, 36, 40, 170–172
survival, 8, 12, 13, 14, 15, 24, 32
　dependent on prenatal conditions, 30–31
　earliest quads, 1–2, 13, 99
　of quintuplets, 23
　　see also Dionne quins
　of sextuplets, 19–21
swaddling, 97 (fig.)
Sweden, quadruplet births in, 112 (table)

185

T

teaching
  effects, 70–71, 71 (table)
  methods, 80–82
time series studies, *see* research methods
training interventions, 9
triplets
  birthweight, 46
  large-scale study, 82–83
  reading studies, 81–82
twin clubs, 86, 170–172
twinning
  mechanism, 33 (fig.)
    in Kaspar quads, 128
  rates, 12
twins
  birthweight, 46
  monochorionic/dichorionic, 47, 79
  monozygotic
    differences between, 76, 89–90, 94
    placentation, 33 (fig.), 115
    similarities, 89
  see also twin studies
Twins and Multiple Births Association, 166, 172
twin studies, 23, 24–25, 42, 47, 52–73 *passim*, 76–94 *passim*
  generalizing to population at large, 88–89
  primary biases in, 87
  T and C (Gesell), 63, 68 (table), 73, 79
  see also research methods

U

ultrasonography, 30
USA, quadruplet births in, 13
uterine inertia, 31

V

Vassilyev, Feodor, 12 (footnote), 96–97 (plate)
visual perception, 57, 59 (figs.)

W

Waddington quins, 21–23
Walton sextuplets, 20 (photo)
We Were Five, 7
'wonderbirths', 17
'Wroclaw quads', 10, 27, 45, 46, 141–142, 142 (photo)
  physical development, 49–51

X

X-ray, 30
  earliest diagnosis of quads, 135
  first diagnosis of quads, 122

Z

zygosity, 1, 3 (fig.), 9, 14–15, 25, 42, 56, 77, 78, 90, 94, 95, 122
  determination, 2, 8, 32–34, 87
    by blood grouping, 34, 52, 116, 139, 145
    by bone ossification, 51–52, 122
    by dermatoglyphics, 128
    by DNA probe, 34
    by footprints, 23
    by physical likeness, 34, 52, 80
    by placental analysis, 28, 31, 32, 33
    by sex, 32
  importance of, 32, 85
  in Dionne quins, 23, 25, 28 (plate)
  in Waddington quins, 23
  influence on birthweight, 47
  possibilities, 3 (fig.)

www.ingramcontent.com/pod-product-compliance
Lightning Source LLC
LaVergne TN
LVHW011001250326
834688LV00003B/53